Social Aspects of HIV

Volume 7

Since the start of the epidemic, HIV and AIDS have fired the imaginations of social as well as medical and public health scientists. This innovative series of books offers a setting in which to publish the very best of social scientific thinking and research. The Social Aspects of HIV series of books offers readers authoritative introductions and overviews, together with summaries of enduring and cutting edge concerns. The series is international and multidisciplinary in focus, including contributions from psychology, sociology, anthropology, education, economic, political and social theory, and international development. Individual volumes offer scholarly overviews of key topics and concerns but also address 'big issues' relevant to HIV prevention, treatment and care. Sexual and drug-related practices; adherence; disclosure; and stigma and discrimination are among topics focused upon, alongside broader cultural, political and social responses to the epidemic, including globalisation and internationalisation. The political economy of AIDS, links to broader questions of sexual health and rights, and the progressive biomedicalisation of the response, will also be among key issues examined. The series will appeal to those working in public health, health psychology, medical sociology, medical anthropology, health promotion, social work and international development. Individual volumes will be relevant to students, teachers, researchers and practitioners within each of these disciplines as well as program developers and managers working across a variety of contexts.

More information about this series at http://www.springer.com/series/11922

Theo Sandfort
Editor

Male Same-sex Sexuality and HIV in Sub-Saharan Africa

Springer

Editor
Theo Sandfort
HIV Center for Clinical and Behavioral Studies
Columbia University and New York State Psychiatric Institute
New York, NY, USA

ISSN 2509-6559 ISSN 2509-6567 (electronic)
Social Aspects of HIV
ISBN 978-3-030-73725-2 ISBN 978-3-030-73726-9 (eBook)
https://doi.org/10.1007/978-3-030-73726-9

This Springer imprint is published by the registered company Springer Nature Switzerland AG.
The registered company address is: Gewerbestrasse 11, 6330 Cham, Switzerland

Preface

This book, *Male Same-sex Sexuality and HIV in Sub-Saharan Africa*, is the outcome of a long journey. That journey started with a working visit to South Africa, at a time, the start of this century, when men who have sex with men in sub-Saharan Africa were nearly completely absent from HIV research. The visit resulted in a working conference aimed at addressing that absence. The proceedings of that conference were aptly called *From Social Silence to Social Science: Perspectives on Same-Sex Sexuality, Gender and HIV/AIDS in South Africa* (Reddy et al., 2009), and the conference led to various research projects focused on HIV. Two more conferences followed, both entitled "African Same-Sex Sexualities and Gender Diversity," which more broadly addressed gender and sexual minority issues in sub-Saharan Africa (Sandfort et al., 2015; Sandfort & Reddy, 2013, 2021).

This journey had several memorable moments. Four such moments illustrate the progress that is possible in a context where same-sex sexuality is so highly stigmatized. The first moment occurred during a visit to a traditional leader in South Africa. The primary role of current traditional leaders, anchored in the South African constitution, is to contribute to the development of society, including the regulation of the social behavior of the people in receipt of their care. The reason for the visit was to obtain the leader's permission to recruit participants for a study of "his people." We were explicit about the purpose of the study and the kind of participants we would like to recruit. To our surprise, he not only gave his permission, but he did also so wholeheartedly without any reservations. In the conversation that followed, he provided a rationale for his response: "These are my people. It is important for me to know about them so that I am better able to take care of them." I can still hear him saying this and, time and again when recalling this incident, his heartfelt words give me goosebumps.

Another moment took place during a meeting with a Community Advisory Board for a study we were about to implement in Malawi. This was a general board meeting, with broad representation of the general community, including a religious leader, a journalist, a teacher, a representative from the police force, and a member of a youth group. We were discussing the relevance of the study. It was clear that the members of the board already had done some work, but there were still some steps to take. "Don't tell us that we have to accept these people," the young person made clear to us. In discussion, the board's arguments moved from statements such as "These men might have sex with our daughters, so to protect our daughters, we better make sure that we know how to prevent HIV transmission in this population" to "These people are people in their own right and deserve to be taken care of." With awe, I witnessed the emotional labor involved in this change of position. A similar trajectory was traveled by a young imam on a Community Advisory Board in Kenya. His initial response to the idea of doing research among men who have sex with men was that these persons should be stoned. That is how he understood Islamic doctrine. Over several months working through various arguments with the other members of the Community Advisory Board, he eventually came around and sincerely and unequivocally supported the study aims.

A fourth experience occurred at the end of one of our studies. We were debriefing some study participants as well as research staff, including nurses, about their experiences during the study. Both the men and the nurses expressed how they had started the study with some hesitations and misgivings. The nurses, who only had their biases to rely upon, were anxious about working with a population they believed they had never met before. Gay and bisexual men were nervous about the kind of treatment they might receive, probably based on prior health service experience. However, by the end of the study, the nurses and men had become best of friends.

Of course, I am not the only one who made this journey. This collection bears witness to the fact that over the past two decades, many scholars, with diverse disciplinary backgrounds, have embarked upon this adventure, all driven by the commitment to eradicate HIV transmission between men, promote appropriate good quality care for men who have sex with men living with HIV, and more generally foster the well-being of sexual minority populations. These scholars have included researchers from countries in sub-Saharan Africa as well as international researchers. They have made visible the disproportionate infection rates, the stigma and discrimination directed toward male same-sex sexuality, but also the opportunities to work with communities to improve health. There is probably no other continent on which working with communities of men who have sex with men is a prerequisite for doing successful research, while empowering the respective communities.

With a focus on male same-sex sexuality, HIV, and sub-Saharan Africa, this book runs the risk of presenting *a single story*: that of men who engage in highly stigmatizing practices, at high risk of HIV infection, and with limited access to appropriate and competent prevention and care. The Nigerian-American novelist, Chimamanda Adichie, warns of the danger of single stories (Adichie, 2009). Such stories reflect only one perspective and run the risk of reinforcing biased assumptions, leading to unbalanced conclusions and decisions, and causing misunderstanding. Such stories can rob people of their dignity, emphasizing differences instead of similarities. "How they are told, who tells them, when they're told, how many stories are told, are really dependent on power," Adichie explains. Given the seriousness of the HIV epidemic, this book's story is important. The account it offers already encapsulates several substories, acknowledging the historical, legal, and cultural differences between sub-Saharan African societies, which affect the expression of same-sex sexuality, the societal response to these practices, as well as the transmission of HIV. But it is important to realize that there are more stories to be told. Despite the stigma and discrimination that they experience, men who have sex with men in sub-Saharan Africa find ways of living. These men have concerns, but also hopes and desires, which go far beyond the risk of HIV.

On a journey, one meets new people and makes new friends. I met many people on my journey and they helped me understand and navigate local cultures. Two of the people I met I would like to mention by name: Vasu Reddy and David Kuria Mbote. My conversations with them helped me better understand the issues that gay, bisexual, and other men who have sex with men face in everyday life. I am grateful to be able to call both of these men my friend. I would like to thank the contributors to this book for entrusting their writing to my editorial efforts. Two other persons need to be thanked for their support in preparing this book: Rebecca Giguere who helped me so conscientiously with the editorial process, and Peter Aggleton who provided substantive feedback on all the chapters and, in doing so, strengthened them. I also thank Peter for his patience, while putting this book together.

This book has been written for all persons in sub-Saharan Africa who express their sexuality and gender in non-normative ways. I hope it will contribute to their health and well-being. It is comforting to know that while, as the figures show, much remains to be accomplished, positive change, however uneven, is beginning to happen.

New York, NY | Theo Sandfort

References

Adichie, C. (2009, July). *The danger of a single story* [Video]. TED Conferences. https://www.ted.com/talks/chimamanda_adichie_the_danger_of_a_single_story

Reddy, V., Sandfort, T., & Rispel, R. (Eds.). (2009). *From social silence to social science: Perspectives on same-sex sexuality, gender and HIV/AIDS in South Africa*. Human Sciences Research Council.

Sandfort, T., & Reddy, V. (Eds.). (2013). African same-sex sexualities and gender diversity. *Culture, Health, and Sexuality, 15*(Suppl 1), S1–S6.

Sandfort, T., & Reddy, V. (Eds.). (2021). African same-sex sexualities and gender diversity. *Sexualities, 24*(1–2), 3–12.

Sandfort, T., Simenel, F., Mwachiro, K., & Reddy, V. (Eds.). (2015). *Boldly queer: African perspectives on same-sex sexuality and gender diversity*. HIVOS.

Contents

Contents

Contributors

Parinita Bhattacharjee Centre for Global Public Health, University of Manitoba, Winnipeg, MB, Canada

Russell Campbell Office of HIV/AIDS Network Coordination, Fred Hutchinson Cancer Research Center, Seattle, WA, USA

Monika Doshi School of Public Health, University of Michigan, Ann Arbor, MI, USA

Daniel K. Gondwe Malawi College of Medicine – Johns Hopkins University Research Project, Blantyre, Malawi

Akua O. Gyamerah University of California, San Francisco, San Francisco, CA, USA

Erica L. Hamilton FHI 360, Durham, NC, USA

Alexander Mwijage Ishungisa Muhimbili University of Health and Allied Sciences, Dar es Salaam, Tanzania

Joshua Kimani Department of Medical Microbiology, University of Nairobi, Nairobi, Kenya

Lisa Lazarus Centre for Global Public Health, University of Manitoba, Winnipeg, MB, Canada

Melkizedeck Thomas Leshabari Muhimbili University of Health and Allied Sciences, Dar es Salaam, Tanzania

Robert Lorway Centre for Global Public Health, University of Manitoba, Winnipeg, MB, Canada

Jonathan Paul Lucas FHI 360, Durham, NC, USA

Pascal Macharia Health Options for Young Men on HIV/AIDS & STIs (HOYMAS), Nairobi, Kenya

John Mathenge Health Options for Young Men on HIV/AIDS & STIs (HOYMAS), Nairobi, Kenya

Tara McKay Vanderbilt University, Nashville, TN, USA

Lyle McKinnon Department of Medical Microbiology, University of Manitoba, Winnipeg, MB, Canada

Brian Minalga Office of HIV/AIDS Network Coordination, Fred Hutchinson Cancer Research Center, Seattle, WA, USA

Elia John Mmbaga Muhimbili University of Health and Allied Sciences, Dar es Salaam, Tanzania

Kåre Moen Department of Community Medicine and Global Health, Institute of Heath and Society, Faculty of Medicine, University of Oslo, Oslo, Norway

Helgar K. Musyoki Kenya National AIDS & STI Control Programme (NASCOP), Ministry of Health, Kenya, Nairobi, Kenya

Akram Pasha Ashodaya Samithi, Mysore, Karnataka, India

Sushena Reza-Paul Centre for Global Public Health, University of Manitoba, Winnipeg, MB, Canada
Ashodaya Samithi, Mysore, Karnataka, India

Theo Sandfort Department of Psychiatry, Columbia University and New York State Psychiatric Institute, New York, NY, USA

Matthew Thomann Department of Anthropology, University of Memphis, Memphis, TN, USA

Chapter 1
Male Same-Sex Sexuality and HIV in Sub-Saharan Africa

Theo Sandfort

To understand the HIV epidemic among men who have sex with men in sub-Saharan Africa, it is vital to appreciate its historical, legal, and social context. While there are differences between Sub-Saharan African countries, related among other things to different experiences of colonization and decolonization, societal acceptance of same-sex sexuality in almost all Sub-Saharan African societies is low. Same-sex practices between men are criminalized in many countries. This context contributes to the invisibility of same-sex sexuality as well as the HIV epidemic among men who have sex with men. In 2012, the overall HIV prevalence among men who have sex with men in sub-Saharan Africa was estimated to be 18%, compared to 5% in all adults which is higher than that for heterosexual men in sub-Saharan Africa (Beyrer et al., 2012). Understanding same-sex sexuality in sub-Saharan Africa requires a closer look at the men engaging in same-sex practices. While in surveys some men may report themselves to be homosexual, gay or bisexual, the local meaning(s) of these labels is less clear. The relatively more frequent transactional sex and the greater bisexual involvement that may be observed among men who have sex with men in sub-Saharan Africa should be understood in the context of societal rejection of same-sex sexuality. With only one in four men living with HIV estimated to be virally suppressed, prevention and care to address the needs of men who have sex with men need to be intensified. This requires initiatives on various levels ranging from working with communities of men who have sex with men, to enabling healthcare systems to deliver appropriate and competent care, to legal reform.

T. Sandfort (✉)
Columbia University and New York State Psychiatric Institute, New York, NY, USA
e-mail: tgs2001@cumc.columbia.edu

T. Sandfort (ed.), *Male Same-sex Sexuality and HIV in Sub-Saharan Africa*, Social Aspects of HIV 7, https://doi.org/10.1007/978-3-030-73726-9_1

1.1 Introduction

"Are there any gay men in Africa?" That was a question I was asked in 2005 by the research manager at a funding institution when I was looking for support for a research project to study HIV transmission between men in South Africa. While the question may have sounded foolish at the time, more than 15 years later, the question is obsolete. A lot more is now known about male same-sex sexuality in sub-Saharan Africa, not the least that sex between men is a major route of HIV transmission on the continent. Our understanding of male same-sex sexuality in sub-Saharan Africa is primarily based on research conducted in the context of HIV. Appraisal of this knowledge requires consideration of the historical, legal, and social context. The epidemiology of HIV offers a compelling explanation for why scholarly attention for men who are having sex with men is warranted. Since the early 2000s, studies in sub-Saharan African countries have demonstrated that the prevalence of HIV among men who have sex with men is substantially higher than among heterosexual men. Research has also given us a better understanding of the diversity within the population of men who have sex with men in terms of their identities, practices and health. Greater awareness of the high HIV prevalence has resulted in the development of national policies (Makofane et al., 2013; WHO, 2018), while international funding has supported the development of community-based organizations. Because of the focus on HIV, other gender and sexual minority groups have received less attention to date, although this may change in the future. Ending the HIV epidemic in sub-Saharan Africa in general, and among men who have sex with men in particular, requires the implementation of supportive policy and further research.

1.2 Historical, Legal, and Social Context

The HIV epidemic among men who have sex with men and male same-sex sexuality itself cannot be understood without considering historical, legal and social contexts in sub-Saharan Africa. While describing these contexts, it is important to keep in mind that sub-Saharan African countries differ in a variety of ways, resulting in part from their distinct histories of colonisation and decolonisation. These differences have implications for the expression of male same-sex sexuality, national responses to HIV among men who have sex with men, and the best way to intervene to reduce stigma and discrimination (Awondo et al., 2012).

Although it has been argued that same-sex sexual practices were imported by traders and colonizers, there is convincing evidence that people in Africa engaged in same-sex sexual practices and that nonbinary gender representations were present well before any contact with Arab traders and Europeans (Epprecht, 2008, 2013; Murray, 2002). This does not imply that precolonial African societies were utopias of sexual freedom. People were expected to have children, but same-sex sexuality could exist alongside heterosexuality in some societies, although not necessarily openly. Sometimes such activities were punished. With colonization in the late nineteenth and early twentieth centuries, however, a "collective silence descended on the topic" according to Epprecht (2013, p. 38). This coincided with a change in conceptions of homosexuality in the Western world: homosexuality was no longer seen as an act, but as a characteristic of a distinct group of people who engaged in these activities, the *homosexuals*. As part of colonization, new settings were created such as mines, prisons, hostels, work camps, industrial ports, and military barracks. These new environments facilitated same-sex sexual relationships, particularly between men.

The criminalization of same-sex sexuality came with the colonizers, especially the British, with maximum sentences ranging from a few years to lifelong imprisonment or death. These laws were applied differently across states and times. Currently, same-sex sexual acts between men are legal in 22 of the 54 African states (Mendos, 2019). In some of these states, same-sex sexual acts have never been criminalized, while in other states, these practices have been decriminalized. In some states where same-sex sexuality is legal, there remains an unequal age of consent for homosexual and heterosexual acts. In other countries same-sex sexuality is not criminalized, but there exists legislation which can be used against persons who engage in same-sex sexual practices. Only one state, South Africa, offers constitutional protection to gay, lesbian, and bisexual people. Over the last 10 years, some countries have drafted laws to increase sanctions against gay, lesbian, and bisexual people, despite of or in reaction to international pressure to decriminalize same-sex sexuality. Overall, however, African states are legally more diverse than generally is thought. Ireland (2013) attributes these differences between states to having, or not, a British colonial past, the presence of a large Muslim population, and the absence of economic freedom and openness.

The legal situation regarding same-sex sexuality is reflected in the social climate in sub-Saharan African countries. In an international review, Lamontagne et al. (2018) concluded that together with the Middle East, Africa is home to the most homophobic countries, South Africa and Cabo Verde being the exceptions. They based their conclusions on a *Homophobic Climate Index*, which assesses the *institutional* and *social* components of homophobia. Institutional homophobia reflects the degree of enforcement of laws that criminalize, protect or recognize same-sex relations. Social homophobia concerns the level of acceptance and justifiability of homosexuality. Higher homophobic climates were observed in countries whose citizens faced gender inequality, human rights abuses, low health expenditures and low life satisfaction. Higher levels of homophobia were also associated with a decrease in the gross domestic product per capita. In terms of health, higher levels of homophobia were associated with increased AIDS-related death among men living with HIV.

Religion plays a critical role in the maintenance of social norms in sub-Saharan Africa, including those regulating sexual practices. In most African societies, religion is deeply integrated into the lives of the people. The ubiquity of religion can be attributed to a cultural and historical legacy that did not sharply distinguish between the sacred and profane. Religion was and still is integrated into the language, culture, and everyday practices of many people (Mbiti, 1990; Selvam & Collicutt, 2013), and religious leaders are often more trusted than other public leaders (Howard, 2020). Most religious leaders adhere to a conservative interpretation of the Bible and other religious texts. So long as theological conservatism remains associated with negative attitudes towards sexual and gender minorities, it is not surprising that religious leader's perspectives are generally negative (Mbote et al., 2018; Stankov & Lee, 2016).

That said, and as has been the case in high-income countries since the mid-twentieth century, a change in attitudes seems to be starting to take place. Between 2002 and 2019, the proportion of people aged 18 years and older, who said that homosexuality should be accepted by society increased in Kenya from 1 to 14%; a similar increase from 1 to 7% occurred between 2013 and 2019 in Nigeria (Poushter & Kent, 2020). Two out of three South Africans support keeping the present protections in the South African Constitution against discrimination on the grounds of sexual orientation. Furthermore, over the past 10 years, there has been a tenfold increase of South Africans who *strongly agree* with allowing same-sex marriage: rising from one in a hundred to one in ten (Sutherland et al., 2016).

1.3 HIV Epidemiology

Some of the first reported cases of HIV infection in sub-Saharan Africa were among white men who had sex with men in South Africa. At the start of the epidemic, cases of HIV seemed to be largely confined to this group (Anderson, 1983; Ras et al., 1983), but they were soon overshadowed by another epidemic with heterosexual sexual intercourse as the dominant mode of transmission. This second epidemic started in Central Africa, involved a different HIV clade (Williamson & Martin, 2005) and resulted in poorer survival rates (Maartens et al., 1997). Black persons were predominantly affected, and women more so than men. As was foreseen from its early identification, the second epidemic turned out to be devastating in its effects (Fleming, 1988). Moreover, the preponderance of heterosexual transmission, combined with the social and cultural invisibility of same-sex sexual practices, concealed the fact that within this generalised epidemic there were concentrated epidemics characterised by same-sex transmission between men.

A first indication of the existence of an HIV epidemic among men who have sex with men in sub-Saharan Africa came from the first HIV prevalence study among men who have sex with men. In this study, conducted in 2004 in Senegal, 21.5% of 463 men who have sex with men tested positive for HIV (Wade et al., 2005). Other studies followed and reported HIV prevalence rates ranging from 4.1 to 49.5% (Baral et al., 2009; Lahuerta et al., 2018; Rispel et al., 2011; Sandfort et al., 2015, 2019; Sullivan et al., 2020; Wirtz et al., 2017). A systematic review conducted in 2012 estimated the overall HIV prevalence among men who have sex with men in sub-Saharan Africa to be 18% (Beyrer et al., 2012). In a review of 17 studies, Hessou et al. (2019) concluded that with an average rate of 17.8% (range: 3.7–33.4) the prevalence of HIV among men who have sex with men was almost five times higher than among men more generally in sub-Saharan Africa. They further observed that prevalence ratios were particularly elevated in West and Central Africa as well as in countries where the overall HIV prevalence was low.

Less is known about the incidence of HIV among men who have sex in sub-Saharan Africa. The few longitudinal studies that have established incidence rates show a range from 5.0 per one-hundred person years (100 PY) (95% CI: 2.5, 10.0) (Couderc et al., 2017) to 15.4/100 PY (95% CI: 12.3, 19.0) (Nowak et al., 2019) (see also Kimani et al., 2019; Lane et al., 2016; Price et al., 2012; Sanders et al., 2013; Sullivan et al., 2020). The observed incidence estimates differed between the four study sites involved in the HIV Prevention Trials Network (HPTN) 075 study, a 1-year prospective biobehavioural cohort study to assess the feasibility of recruiting and retaining men who have sex with men. These incidence rates were: 1.3/100 PY in Blantyre (Malawi), 3.8/100 PY in Kisumu (Kenya), 9.0/100 PY in Soweto (South Africa), and 14.4/100 PY in Cape Town (South Africa) (Sandfort et al., 2021). These incidence estimates are substantially higher than those reported for the year 2017 in 15–49 years old persons in general in the respective countries (0.17%, 0.45%, and 0.86% for Kenya, Malawi, and South Africa, respectively) (Joint United Nations Programme on HIV/AIDS, 2020).

These prevalence and incidence estimates should be treated with caution. Although several studies used respondent-driven sampling as recruitment strategy to enhance the sample, other studies did not, making it difficult to generalise from the findings. Furthermore, when comparing prevalence and incidence, one should be aware that variations in these estimates reflect real population differences as well as differences in study design. For instance, studies that have strict eligibility criteria that lead to the selection of men with disproportionately high sexual risk will tend to report higher prevalence and incidence rates than studies that apply less strict inclusion criteria.

The presented incidence rates make clear that men who have sex with men in sub-Saharan Africa are at extremely high risk for HIV infection. However, the data do not inform us about the current status of the epidemic among men who have sex with men. Is the epidemic among men who have sex with men under control or is transmission still increasing? The few available data do not make one optimistic. A study in Nigeria, using respondent-driven sampling as a recruitment strategy to approach population estimates, showed a consistent and significant increase in HIV prevalence among men who have sex with men with about 10-percentage points relative increase per year over a 7-year period from 2007 to 2014 (Eluwa et al., 2019).

1.4 Sexual Identities

Addressing HIV among men who have sex with men in sub-Saharan Africa requires a close understanding of the population concerned. Most research studies among men who have sex with men describe the sexual identities of the persons in their samples as *gay* or *bisexual*. This descriptive information is often provided in a self-evident way, as if the meaning of these labels is unambiguous, and as if it is clear how these persons understand themselves in terms of their sexuality and what the sexual and identity practices are that they engage in. This is also true for the more general term *men who have sex with men*. Although this label may be relevant from a narrow epidemiological perspective, it tells us very little about the sexual realities of the persons involved and, as we will see later in this book, the label men who have sex with men covers a very diverse set of individuals, practices and circumstances. Understanding these realities is critical if one wants to support men to protect their health and promote well-being.

Because the world has become smaller and more interconnected, it is likely that the words "gay" and "bisexual" have become part of many of the vocabularies in societies across sub-Saharan Africa. That does not mean though that everybody in these societies is familiar with these words. Even men who have sex with men may not know or identify with these labels. It also does not mean that everybody familiar with these terms understands them in a similar way and that this understanding is identical to how the labels are understood in high income countries.

Misunderstandings, or better, idiosyncratic understandings of what these labels mean are illustrated by what some of the participants said about their identities in the HPTN 075 study referred to above (Sandfort et al., 2020). A 24-year-old man in Kenya first indicated in a survey that he was bisexual and sexually attracted to both men and women. Later, in an interview, he said he was *gay*. When discussing what is meant by the term "men who have sex with men," he said: "I think the *gay* fits in that MSM [men who have sex with men] community, because they are not bisexual. I think also bisexual can do, but the most popular in the community are the gay." Curious about the use of the word *bisexual* here, the interviewer asked: "What do you mean by bisexual?" In response, the man said "I think bisexual, these are people in a community who have two sexual organs. That is the penis and the vagina." In the same study, a young bisexual man in Malawi said, "A person who is gay, according to me, is a person that looks like a girl that has feelings towards men." A young South African person, asked what it was that made them say that they were gay, responded: "... Because I like boys. Everything about me, like, I feel like a girl, actually, just in a man's body. So, I'm attracted to boys mostly physically, spiritually, like yeah." When, in the same study, a young person who identified as *female* was asked what kind of persons would fit the category men who have sex with men, they responded: "Straight men. (...) Yes, because you cannot get the gay man and another gay man sleeping together. It's hardly possible. (...) As you see me, I'm like a sister, like a girl. So, I cannot go to another person who looks like me. (...) I'm going for a maaaaaan. Like a real man!"

This focus on the labels *gay* and *bisexual* ignores the fact that English is the official language in only a very few of the 46 sub-Saharan countries. Furthermore, in countries where English is the official language, it is not the only one and most often only spoken by a small segment of the population. For instance, English is the official language in Zimbabwe, but the first language of only around 2% of the population (Shona and Ndebele are spoken by most of the population). In Nigeria, over 500 languages are spoken. While English is the country's official language, other languages, including Hausa, Igbo, Yoruba, Efik, Edo, Adamawa, Fulfulde, Idoma, and Central Kanuri, are all widely spoken.

This rich linguistic diversity combined with the precolonial presence of same-sex sexuality is reflected in the existence of indigenous words characterising same-sex sexual practices or the person who engage in these practices (Leap, 2004; Moen et al., 2014; Porter, 1995; Thompson, 2015). This diversity is rarely acknowledged in HIV-related research. An exception is a study among Kenyan men who have sex with men which described men as identifying, among others, as *basha*, *hanithi*, *kuchu*, and *shoga* (Quilter et al., 2019), albeit without explaining what the meaning of these somewhat different local labels was. Basha is a Swahili word used by men to indicate that they primarily engage in anal sex in the insertive role. Hanithi has its origins in Arabic and is used for men who have the receptive role in anal sex. Shoga in Swahili is the main word for gay person, male or female, but is also used to refer to a very good female friend and as an adjective to denote behaving in a way that is associated with women. The exact meanings of such indigenous labels are likely to differ by society. Some of these meanings may be derogatory, and it is not clear whether the adoption of such derogatory labels is an indication of internalized shame or whether they have been reappropriated and adopted as an indication of resistance. The latter is definitely the case with the traditionally prejorative term kuchu, an equivalent of the English word *queer*, as used within the Uganda LGBT community. This label gained popularity through the documentary *Call me Kuchu* (https://callmekuchu.com) which showed the oppressive situation in which lesbian, gay, and bisexual people in Uganda live. Other African societies have other labels with complex historical and indigenous origins.

Little is known about how men come to adopt certain sexual identity labels or more generally about sexual identity development among men who have sex with men in sub-Saharan Africa (see however Gyamerah et al., 2019). This gap in understanding should be understood in the context of intense stigma and, in some countries, criminalisation, which complicates visibility and the developmental process. This context makes it harder to develop a sense of what it means to experience same-sex attraction and to find out how to express these feelings. It also makes it harder to find information about same-sex sexuality, relationships and practices. With less visibility, it will be more difficult to find role-models or like-minded people. There will be lack of support from one's direct environment, while expressions of same-sex sexuality are likely to be ostracised and rejected. Such challenging development processes are likely to have long-term implications for individual and community well-being and health.

1.5 Sexual Practices

Relatively late awareness and acknowledgment that men who have sex with men in sub-Saharan Africa engage in sexual practices that put them at risk for HIV infection, has over the past two decades produced a flurry of studies mapping these men's sexual behaviour. As with questions about sexual identification, these studies tell only part of the story, by not putting behaviour into a broader context. Nevertheless, men's reports about their behaviours already highlight particularities that are important to understand in the context of HIV prevention. One such specificity seems to be that as far as men engage in anal sex, they do so more exclusively as either the insertive or receptive partner, in comparison to men who have sex with men in high income countries. For instance, among men who have sex with men in Kenya, 29% reported having engaged in both insertive and receptive anal sex in the preceding 3 months (Sanders et al., 2007). Based on lifetime behaviour, 34% of the men who have sex with men in South Africa reported having engaged in both insertive and receptive anal sex (Sandfort et al., 2015). In a study among men who have sex with men in California, 55% of the men reported having engaged in both insertive and receptive anal sex in the preceding 6 months (Wei & Raymond, 2011), whereas, on a 1-year basis, this proportion was 83% among men in an Australian study (Lyons et al., 2011).

The few attempts that have been made to understand these behavioural patterns suggest the role of two related factors. The first is that men with more feminine modes of gender expression are more likely to engage in receptive anal intercourse, whereas men with more masculine forms of expression are more likely to engage in insertive anal sex. Second, men who see themselves as more masculine are also more likely to have sex with women. It is possible that in sub-Saharan Africa male same-sex sexual practices are more structured around gender roles than they are in high income countries. Regardless, the HIV epidemic among men who have sex with men in sub-Saharan Africa would likely be even more severe than the current data indicate if there was more sexual role versality (Cortés, 2018; Wiley & Herschkorn, 1989). The protective impact of role separation is likely to be undermined by other structural factors that hinder the adoption of safer sex practices in sub-Saharan Africa. Still, better insight in sexual role separation may help strengthen the support available to men with receptive versus insertive anal sex preferences when adopting and maintaining safer sex practices.

1.5.1 Transactional Sex and Sex Work

Another feature of sexual behaviour among men who have sex with men in sub-Saharan Africa is the seemingly high proportion of men who engage in transactional sex. For instance, in a study of a population-based sample of men who have sex with men in Nairobi, Kenya, an estimated proportion of 40% of men had sold sex in the preceding 2 months or reported *sex work* as their main occupation (Muraguri et al., 2015). If the study had looked at the broader category of transactional sex, which also includes sex in exchange for things other than money and in which money is not necessarily the driving motive, this proportion would likely have been higher.

Engagement in transactional sex has often been seen as a risk factor for HIV infection. An overview of studies suggests that although not on other continents, this is indeed the case for men who have sex with men in sub-Saharan Africa, as well as in Latin America (Oldenburg et al., 2015). Because most studies about transactional sex among men who have sex with men have used cross-sectional study designs, it is not clear whether sex work in and of itself explains the increased prevalence. Other factors are likely to play a role as well. For instance, Muraguri et al. (2015) found that men who engage in sex work not only report a higher number of receptive anal sex partners and unprotected anal sex, but also increased exposure to various types of abuse or assault, which may compound their risk. Engagement in sex work may also limit access to HIV prevention.

Even though financial hardship is an important driver of why men sell sex to other men (Duncan et al., 2017), it is important to consider the broader social context. Reliance on transactional sex may be a consequence of limited access to regular employment due to high levels of stigma and discrimination. In an environment where same-sex sexuality is highly stigmatised, sex may also become a rare and sought-after commodity, increasing its economic value. It is possible that with an increased acceptance of same-sex sexuality, the prevalence of transactional sex among men will diminish.

Research on transactional sex among men who have sex with men in sub-Saharan Africa has predominantly focused on persons receiving money or other benefits whereas the men who providing the money or resources remain out of the picture. Kounta et al. (2019) showed in a cohort study among men who have sex with men in Burkina Faso, Côte d'Ivoire, Mali, and Togo, that most clients adopted HIV risk reduction strategies, including engaging in protected anal sex, avoidance of sex when consuming psychoactive products, and practising exclusively insertive anal sex. It is not clear, however, whether the male clients in this study were representative of men who pay other men for sex. Another study, in which clients were recruited through peer educators, identified various barriers to safer sex in male sex work interactions, including extra-payment for condomless sex, low perceived HIV/STI risk with some sexual partners, perceived reduced pleasure associated with using condoms, alcohol use, and violence towards male sex workers by clients (Valente et al., 2020).

1.5.2 Sex with Men and Women

Studies of sexual behaviour of men who have sex with men in sub-Saharan Africa also show that compared to men in high income countries, relatively large proportions of men also have sex with women. This difference is not only present when one looks at lifetime behaviour, but also when more recent time periods are considered. For instance, in a study among 557 Nigerian men who have sex with men, 48% had also engaged in sex with women in the previous 2 months (Sheehy et al., 2014). In an earlier study, Beyrer et al. (2010) reported that more than half of 537 men who have sex with men in Malawi, Namibia and Botswana had also had sex with women in the preceding 6 months, while one third of them were married or had a regular female partner.

Men who have sex with both men and women seem to differ in various ways from men who only have sex with men. There are of course differences in sexual attraction and identity in line with the differences in behaviour, with behaviourally bisexual men being more likely to report that they also experience sexual attraction to women and adopt the label bisexual or straight. These men also differ in terms of how they deal with same-sex attraction; they report relatively less positive feelings about same-sex attraction and disclose these feelings less frequently. There are also differences in terms of sexual behaviour. Men who have sex with men and women are more likely to be the insertive partner in anal sex, and potentially in relation to this, are less likely to be HIV positive. In addition, these men seem more likely to pay for sex instead of being paid, in comparison with men who only have sex with men (Alcala-Alezones et al., 2018; Beyrer et al., 2010; Sheehy et al., 2014).

There are several ways in which to understand the relatively high prevalence of bisexual behaviour among men who have sex with men in sub-Saharan Africa. First, it may be that there are relatively more men who experience sexual attraction to both men and women. Such feelings could be induced by legal and cultural influences discouraging same-sex behaviour. It is more likely that for some men, engaging in sex with women or adopting a heterosexual lifestyle is a way to hide one's same-sex practices and conform to local standards. The importance of social context is supported by findings from the HPTN 075 study. The study found that in South Africa, were same-sex sexuality is legal and sexual orientation is protected in the Constitution, bisexual behaviour was reported to be less prevalent among men who have sex with men than in Malawi and Kenya, where same-sex sexuality is criminalised (Ondeng'e et al., 2018). The pressure to adopt a heterosexual lifestyle should also be understood in relation to the importance of procreation to endow status and ensure lineage (Epprecht, 2006). If procreation is the reason for engaging in sex with a woman, condom use is unlikely (Larmarange et al., 2010).

One might speculate about what might happen to these behavioural patterns in the future. Will all gay men in sub-Saharan Africa become behaviourally bisexual as they get older, which seems to be suggested by the fact that in studies men who have sex with men in sub-Saharan Africa are rarely older than 35? Or, if the social context is critical and social acceptance of same-sex sexuality increases, will young men who come out now be less likely to adopt a heterosexual lifestyle, suggesting that a bisexual or heterosexual lifestyle is more a generational phenomenon?

The relatively high prevalence of sex with women among men who have sex with men in sub-Saharan Africa has important implications for understanding the HIV epidemic and for ways of preventing the onward transmission of HIV. Yet, little work is being done to understand the epidemiological implications of the high prevalence of bisexual behaviour. There is little to no HIV prevention programming that takes into account the specific needs of men who have sex with both men and women in sub-Saharan Africa. There is also no discussion of the implications for women of having sex with men who have sex with men.

1.6 Beyond Sexual Behaviour

Given that it was the HIV epidemic that instigated the growth of research into men who have sex with men in sub-Saharan Africa, it is understandable that the primary focus has been on men's sexual behaviour. Existing studies provide important insights into how men's sexual practices are structured and the context of these practices and, as such, inform HIV prevention strategies. As in high-income countries, sexual risk is often associated with a variety of psychosocial adversity factors, including lack of knowledge of HIV, stigma, childhood adversity, intimate partner violence, food insecurity and depressive symptoms, that may reinforce each other (Coulaud et al., 2020; Essack et al., 2020; Nelson et al., 2015; Oginni et al., 2019; Ogunbajo et al., 2020; Okafor et al., 2018; Sandfort et al., 2013b). Yet another set of factors relates to the role of substance use in engagement with unprotected sex behaviours.

1.6.1 Substance Use

A review of 68 studies among men who have sex with men in sub-Saharan Africa, mainly conducted in countries where Christianity is the predominant religion, showed that the use of alcohol and drugs has mostly been studied in association with the use of protection in sexual interactions (Sandfort et al., 2017). Most of these studies looked at the amount of substance use and its relationship with engagement in unprotected or condomless sex.

The frequency of alcohol and drug use varies across studies, however. Some studies reported substantial proportions of men engaging in hazardous drinking, whereas in other studies alcohol use was comparatively lower. These differences likely reflect geographic and cultural differences between African countries (Woolf-King et al., 2013). Comparisons with rates of alcohol use in various African countries provided by the WHO (2014) suggest, however, that across African countries alcohol use is more prevalent among men who have sex with men than men in general.

Levels of drug use among men who have sex with men also varied between countries, although overall drugs seemed to be used much less often than alcohol. If drug use is reported, it is usually cannabis that is mentioned. In general, injection drug use is low across Africa compared with other parts of the world—for 2017, the estimated proportion of persons in Africa who injected drugs was 0.12%, compared with 0.55% in Europe and 0.62% in North America (United Nations Office of Drugs and Crime, 2019). However, studies in Malawi, Namibia, Nigeria, and Tanzania, do report a relatively high prevalence of injection drug use among men who have sex with men (Adebajo et al., 2014; Baral et al., 2009; Johnston et al., 2010; Sanders et al., 2007).

As in research conducted among African populations in general (Hahn et al., 2011) as well as in non-Africa–based studies (Maisto & Simons, 2016), use of alcohol or drugs is associated with engagement in HIV risk behaviours among men who have sex with men in sub-Saharan Africa. In addition, alcohol and drug use is associated with various other risk factors for HIV infection, including experiences of violence and transactional sex. Inconsistent with other research, though, studies rarely found an association between substance use and HIV infection. Many men who reported having sex under the influence of alcohol or drugs seem to be aware that having sex under the influence increases their risk (King et al., 2013; Okall et al., 2013). The fact that substance use is not always associated with condomless sex suggests that some men adopt protective strategies that may work even when under the influence of substances consumed.

In qualitative studies of men who have sex with men in sub-Saharan Africa, substance use is reported to facilitate social and sexual interactions, reinforce sexual desire, induce sexual disinhibition, reduce self-efficacy, and lead to poor decision-making (Musinguzi et al., 2015; Okal et al., 2009). This seems similar to what is reported by persons who engage in heterosexual sex. Reasons why substance use may be relatively more salient to men who have sex with men derive from the fact that it can be used to reduce the pain associated with being the receptive partner in anal sex, to help overcome the stigma that is often associated with same-sex sexuality, or because drinking establishments are often one of the few possible locations for men to meet sexual partners. Substance use may also be associated with sexual risk factors that are more specific to men who have sex with men, such as multiple partnerships, sex in public places, group sex, transactional sex, sexual coercion, symptoms of rectal trauma, and concurrent STIs.

1.7 Prevention, Care, and Treatment Cascade

It is not clear whether the HIV epidemic among men who have sex with men in sub-Saharan Africa is under control and, in particular, whether HIV incidence is increasing or decreasing. The observed prevalence of HIV suggests the need to intensify HIV prevention and pre-exposure prophylaxis (PrEP) could be a critical addition to the available strategies (Couderc et al., 2017). While there seems to be strong interest in PrEP among men who have sex with men in several sub-Saharan African countries (Coulaud et al., 2018; Kimani et al., 2019), there may be adherence challenges (Kimani et al., 2021). With careful attention to uptake and adherence, PrEP could have a major impact on HIV transmission between men who have sex with men in sub-Saharan Africa. The role of PrEP should not be overstated, though. Apart from the fact the PrEP might not always be the preferred prevention tool and the observed PrEP adherence problems (Wahome et al., 2020), it is important to realize that PrEP does not address other barriers to the adoption of safer sex practices, such as criminalisation and stigmatisation. PrEP can only be one element in the strategy to end the HIV epidemic among sub-Saharan African men who have sex with men.

More is understood about HIV testing, engagement in care, the uptake of antiretroviral therapy (ART), and viral suppression. A systematic review and meta-analysis of 75 studies, including a total number of 44.993 men who had sex with men, demonstrates some important trends, but also points at major gaps, requiring further research (Stannah et al., 2019). The findings themselves demonstrate the urgency of invigorated HIV prevention activities as well as the need for structural change. Using pooled estimates, over 60% of all men in these studies had ever tested for HIV; with 46%, the proportion of men who tested in the preceding year being only one quarter smaller. Both proportions have increased regularly over time. However, that more HIV testing and repeat HIV testing is needed, is suggested by the small proportion of men who are HIV positive and aware of their status, which, estimated across studies to be 18%, is very low. This estimate suggests that four out of five men who have sex with men and who are living with HIV in sub-Saharan Africa are not aware of their HIV status, a proportion that has not changed in the past 10 years. Findings regarding engagement in care, receiving ART, and being virally suppressed are even less encouraging. According to the review of Stannah et al. (2019), 40% of men who are living with HIV are currently in receipt of care, but only one in seven men was linked to care within 30 days of diagnosis. About one quarter of the men who were living with HIV were on ART; a proportion which doubled if one only looks at men who are aware of their HIV positive status. The estimates regarding viral suppression that Stannah and colleagues present are telling. Of all men who were living with HIV, regardless of whether they were aware of their status, about 25% were virally suppressed. This is 34% among men who were aware of their positive HIV status. Among men who currently are on ART, 76% is estimated to be virally suppressed. This latter percentage indicates that once on ART, many men can reach viral suppression and consequently lower the risk of onward transmission (see also Palumbo et al., 2021).

The same review explored how indicators of the HIV treatment cascade varied between countries in relation to the law regarding same-sex sexuality. The role of four key indicators was explored: the existence of repressive legislation (e.g., sexual orientation-related non-governmental organisations are illegal, age of consent differs for same-sex relationships); the absence of protective legislation (e.g., incitement to hatred based on sexual orientation is not illegal); the absence of progressive legislation (e.g., same-sex marriage is not legally recognised); and the level of punishment received for consensual same-sex sexual interactions, varying from no punishment to the death penalty. The study found negative associations between the severity of legislation with HIV testing and HIV status awareness. The more severe legislation was the less HIV testing and awareness of a positive HIV status were observed. It is likely that in a (potentially) more punitive environment, men who have sex with men will be less likely to come out to healthcare providers or engage in care. This could result from negative feelings men have about their same-sex behaviour, expectations of stigmatising treatment or actual negative experiences, lack of trust regarding confidential treatment, or doubts about presence of appropriate expertise. Importantly, in such a context the healthcare system may not be able to deliver appropriate care in a non-stigmatising way.

Comparing treatment cascade indicators with those from men who have sex with men living on other continents, the review suggests that the situation for men who have sex with men in sub-Saharan Africa is worse. Furthermore, the overall picture for men who have sex with men differs markedly from that pertaining to men in general. The proportion of men who have sex with men who test for HIV is consistently higher compared to other men across regions in sub-Saharan Africa. Nevertheless, awareness of living with HIV and being on ART is substantially lower among men who have sex with men.

1.8 Healthcare Access: Challenges and Facilitators

Given the limited acceptance of same-sex sexuality in sub-Saharan Africa, and its criminalisation in some countries, it is not surprising that healthcare options for persons engaging in same-sex sexuality are suboptimal. The diverse barriers to healthcare access that are faced by men who have sex with men have been documented in several studies. These barriers exist on top of the difficulties that people in general experience in accessing healthcare within the region (Babalola & Moodley, 2020). Most existing research has focused on the experiences of men who have sex with men with healthcare. Men report concerns about privacy and confidentiality, and inadequate care and negative healthcare experiences, including various forms of abuse from providers (Magesa et al., 2014; Wanyenze et al., 2016; Wirtz et al., 2014). In a cross-national study, almost half of the participants in Kenya, Malawi and South Africa reported at least one healthcare-related stigma experience (Mbeda et al., 2020). The most frequently reported experiences included fear of seeking healthcare services and avoiding seeking such services because of the potential discovery of involvement in same-sex practices. However, few participants reported actually having been denied health services because of having sex with men. Healthcare stigma experiences were more likely among men who experienced less social support or who reported that they did not have friends and a supportive community to rely on.

1.8.1 Disclosure and Healthcare Providers Responses

Receiving care for health issues related to one's same-sex sexual identity and/or practices requires disclosure to healthcare providers. Non-disclosure may result in misdiagnosis and prescription of inappropriate treatment. Such disclosure may elicit various negative responses from healthcare providers, including rejection or the refusal of services. Men's experiences of healthcare seem to vary, partly based on their sense of agency. For instance, Lane et al. (2008) observed that among men who have sex with men in South Africa, sexual health-seeking practices differ according to sexual and gender identification. Men who identified as gay and who were more likely to be gender nonconforming, would confront healthcare workers when they encountered homophobia and claim their rights to obtain non-stigmatising health services. The men who identified as bisexual or straight were more likely to avoid disclosing their practices and accentuate their masculine identity when presenting for sexual health services, thereby risking not receiving the care that they needed.

Because of their education and training informed by heteronormative curricula, healthcare providers often lack the clinical skills to perform basic functions, such as the diagnosis of anal sexually transmitted infections (Rebe et al., 2019). Moreover, the challenges that men who have sex with men experience in accessing healthcare do not stand on their own since healthcare access-related barriers are reflective of broader societal rejection of same-sex sexuality. For instance, in a study among men who have sex with men in Burkina Faso, Kim et al. (2018) found that ever being afraid of or avoiding health care services—reported by 25% of 330 men—because someone might find out about their engagement in sex with other men, was associated with stigma more generally, experiencing verbal harassment and feeling scared to walk in public.

1.8.2 Care for Men Who Have Sex with Men Who Are Living with HIV

The problem of access to appropriate and competent healthcare is particularly severe for men who have sex with men who are living with HIV. This is clearly illustrated by the fact that in sub-Saharan Africa, only one in four of such men is estimated to be virally suppressed (Stannah et al., 2019). Balogun et al. (2020) explored the barriers experienced by men who have sex with men living with HIV in Nigeria, where same-sex practices are criminalised. Their analysis showed that men encountered two main barriers in accessing healthcare facilities: barriers relating to the wider societal context and barriers directly related to services.

Wider contextual barriers include aspects of society that make it difficult for men to access healthcare services freely, including the criminalisation of same-sex sexuality. Barriers regarding access to services include lack of confidentiality and the fear or actual experience that information about one's sexual behaviour and/or HIV status will be shared outside the clinic. Yet another barrier derived from the stigmatising and discriminatory attitudes of providers, leading in some cases to the denial of medical treatment. The expectation that providers will lack the competence to address health problems specific to men who have sex with men was also mentioned.

Additional barriers were more general and likely to be experienced by other people as well. These more general barriers included the preferential treatment afforded to prominent clients or clients who healthcare providers knew, the need to pay bribes or inducements in order to access services, overcrowding, long queues and long waiting times. Having to receive care in separate wards labelled HIV was also experienced as stigmatizing. A few men who have sex with men also reported the existence of friendly healthcare facilities. Such facilities were sparse, though, and quite often far from where men lived, which created a challenge but, because of the associated anonymity, was also a facilitator (Balogun et al., 2020).

Similar barriers have been reported elsewhere by other researchers such as Ogunbajo et al. (2018) in Ghana. Here, factors that influenced engagement in HIV care included fear of mortality from HIV, knowledge of the effectiveness of HIV treatment, enrolment in health insurance, having had positive experiences in the healthcare setting, and prior relationships and familiarity with hospital personnel. Another facilitator was social support from individuals who motivated and encouraged men to seek and sustain treatment. These persons included family members and friends, but also relationships that materialized because of an HIV diagnosis. Some of the support provided included information about the benefits of HIV medications and possible detrimental outcomes of avoiding treatment. Nurses and doctors sometimes played a major role in encouraging men to stay in care.

The barriers to care engagement and antiretroviral therapy adherence experienced by men who have sex with men and are living with HIV are not unknown to healthcare providers. In interviews with Kenyan healthcare providers, Micheni et al. (2017) found common challenges such as HIV-related stigma and lack of disclosure, but the providers also noted challenges that were specific to men who have sex with men, which included economic and social inequality due to stigma, difficult relationships with care providers, and discrimination both at the clinic and in the community.

1.8.3 Alternative Strategies

What do men who have sex with men do if they experience significant barriers to access but need healthcare? Some men avoid seeking care and leave concerns such as a suspected STI untreated. Others seek to obtain medications directly from pharmacies or drugstores. Agardh et al. (2017) interviewed 15 men who have sex with men in Dar es Salaam, who had sought assistance relating to their sexual health at pharmacies and drugstores. Their choice of pharmacies and drugstores was informed by concerns about privacy and confidentiality in healthcare facilities, often based on actual negative experiences. These threats were set against physical symptoms that indicated an increasing need for treatment. Men used their social networks to locate pharmacists who were willing to help, were not judgemental, and did not ask questions. Actual experiences were not always positive, though. Some pharmacists were business oriented. The men did not always fully trust the services that they received and, on some occasions, the services provided turned out to be insufficient. While in some situations, pharmacies may offer a viable alternative to formal healthcare for some health problems, education is needed for men who have sex with men as well as pharmacists. In relation to the treatment of STIs, such education should include the risks of antibiotic resistance.

1.8.4 Moving Forward

Addressing the HIV epidemic among men who have sex with men in sub-Saharan Africa requires the creation of an enabling social and political environment in which men who have sex with men can freely access healthcare services and receive competent care. Various recommendations have been made to improve access to healthcare (Micheni et al., 2017; Rebe et al., 2019). They include the development and implementation of best practice guidelines, better education for healthcare providers, clinic staff sensitivity training, the use of trained peer navigators, broad stakeholder engagement, and the use of community engagement strategies and social media technologies. Only addressing individual barriers is likely to be insufficient. Multilevel interventions are necessary to engage with structural factors to promote and reinforce sustained change in healthcare settings.

There are indications of the kind of strategies that might work. For instance, Van der Elst et al. (2013) assessed the effect of a web-based, self-directed sensitivity training on same-sex sexuality for healthcare workers in four districts of coastal Kenya (www.marps-africa.org). They combined the course with facilitated group discussion among healthcare workers from 49 health facilities. Three months after the intervention, knowledge of sexual health needs had significantly improved compared to before the intervention. Furthermore, homophobic attitudes had significantly decreased 3 months after training. Improvement of knowledge seemed to be associated with a reduction in homophobic feelings.

Lyons et al. (2017) evaluated the impact of a 3-tiered integrated stigma mitigation intervention approach to optimizing HIV service delivery for key populations (men who have sex with men and female sex workers) in Senegal. The three tiers included a community level intervention to target perceived stigma, a clinical level intervention to address enacted stigma by healthcare workers, and, at a post-clinical level, a peer-to-peer web-based referral system using social media to assist key populations in locating non-stigmatizing health services. The impact of the approach was evaluated in a cohort of men who have sex with men through the uptake of HIV services and implementation outcomes. Fear of seeking health services decreased significantly among men. However, men felt that enacted stigma from health workers that impeded access to care did not improve. More work is clearly needed to understand how to implement competent and appropriate care optimally for men who have sex with men.

1.9 Other Sexual and Gender Minorities

Disproportionate rates of HIV infection are the main reason why research among sexual and gender minorities in sub-Saharan Africa has primarily focused on men. Compared to men who have sex with men, other sexual and gender minority groups have received much less research attention. However, a body of research is emerging focused on transgender women, again prompted by the HIV epidemic. While transgender women were initially included in studies focused on men who have sex with men, they have started receiving independent scholarly attention (Cloete et al., 2019). The relative unlikelihood of HIV transmission between women has stymied research among women who have sex with women, although findings from a few studies indicate that HIV is a matter of concern within this population. Likewise, there has been little or no research on men with non-binary identifications or the multitude of romantic and other minority gender and sexual identifications now widely used in the social media and other contexts, among young people in particular (Cover, 2018, 2020). Recent efforts to distinguish between romantic and sexual attraction, for example, complicate understanding of the affective dimensions of gender and sexuality as they relate to men, some of whom engage in same sex practices (Diamond, 2004); this distinction may be of relevance in the context of sub-Saharan Africa in helping the understand men who engage in sex with men and women. Given the important opportunities that social media offer in the process of discovering one's sexual and gender status (Szulc & Dhoest, 2013), especially in a context where gender and sexual diversity are stigmatized, it is likely that these diverse gender and sexual identifications also will be adopted in sub-Saharan Africa. The implications of this expansion for HIV research, prevention and care still must be explored, in sub-Saharan Africa as well as in other parts of the world, including high-income countries.

1.9.1 Transgender Persons

There are several possible reasons why transgender women were initially included in HIV-related research focused on men who have sex men in sub-Saharan Africa. With limited access to transgender role models, coming out as transgender may be slowed and start with a provisional identification as gay, because of a shared desire for sex with men (Sandfort et al., 2018). It is also possible that some persons identify as female, based on their strong preference of receptive anal sex. In a strong heteronormative context in which gender roles are separated, this preference may lead these persons to see themselves and be seen by others as women, without them having the desire to undergo any modifications to align their body with the experienced gender (Essack et al., 2020; Sandfort et al., 2018). Some transgender women in sub-Saharan Africa identify as *gay* or see themselves as part of a gay community (Sandfort et al., 2018). This integration may be similar to the early stages in the history of the transgender movement in other countries, when the boundaries between non-heteronormative gender and sexual groups were less strictly defined (Minter, 2000). In some studies, transgender women were included based on community input and the desire to be inclusive and respectful of how local communities define themselves (Sandfort et al., 2020).

As research in other parts of the world have shown, transgender women in sub-Saharan Africa are at increased risk of HIV infection. In three South African cities, an HIV prevalence of 50 to 73% has been recorded among trans women (Cloete et al., 2019) and in Nairobi, an HIV prevalence of 41% has been identified (Smith et al., 2021). In the HPTN 075 study, transgender women in Kenya, Malawi and South Africa had an odds ratio for HIV infection of 2.02 (CI 95%: 1.36, 3.01) compared to cisgender men have sex with men (Sandfort et al., 2019). Other studies report similar findings (Keshinro et al., 2016; Poteat et al., 2017; Smith et al., 2021; Stahlman et al., 2016). When it comes to HIV incidence among trans women much less is known. The HPTN 075 study found an incidence of 8.4/100 person-years (PY) (95% CI: 2.3, 21.5) among trans women (Sandfort et al., 2021).

Little is also known about trans women in relation to the HIV prevention, treatment, and care cascade. In a national study in Kenya, only 17% of the trans persons who reported being HIV positive were in receipt of treatment (Trans*Alliance et al., 2020). As with men who have sex with men, the elevated risk of HIV infection among trans women in countries such as the USA has been shown to be linked to a combination of multi-level factors (Mimiaga et al., 2019; Operario & Nemoto, 2010; Poteat et al., 2016b), including childhood sexual abuse, substance use, intimate partner violence, depression, parental rejection, antitransgender stigma and transgender specific victimization, and economic hardship. Although a similar scenario may prevail in sub-Saharan Africa, studies specifically focused on transgender women are rare. About transgender men and HIV in sub-Saharan Africa even less is known.

Although the inclusion of transgender women in HIV-related research focused on men who have sex with men has provided some important insights, this practice is also deeply problematic. To start with, even when transgender women are included, results are not always disaggregated, leaving the specific needs of transgender women hard to discern (Poteat et al., 2016a; Sevelius et al., 2016). Furthermore, with men who have sex with men being the focus of these studies, assessment tools may not align with the experiences of transgender women or leave their needs unaddressed. Finally, comparison with men who have sex with men perpetuates the notion that transgender women are men, and not women. It is obvious that elevated HIV prevalence among transgender women in SSA warrants studying the health needs of this population in its own right.

1.9.2 Women Who Have Sex with Women

The general assumption that sexual transmission of HIV between women is rare has led to the misunderstanding that women who have sex with women are not at risk for HIV infection. In consequence, lesbian and bisexual women have long been overlooked by HIV research and programming (Cloete et al., 2011). A few studies have explored HIV infection among women who have sex with women in sub-Saharan Africa (Tat et al., 2015). Unlike most research among men who have sex with men, these studies have depended on the self-report of HIV infection, quite likely resulting in a serious underestimation of actual prevalence. Among

591 women who have sex with women from Botswana, Namibia, South Africa, and Zimbabwe, 10% reported to be living with HIV (Sandfort et al., 2013a); and living with HIV was more likely among women who reported to ever had experienced forced sex. In Lesotho, 8% of 208 women who have sex with women (Poteat et al., 2014) reported living with HIV and having a positive HIV status was associated with reporting to have had three or more male sexual partners or sexual partners of both sexes in the preceding year, and with a history of sexually transmitted infections. In these and other studies of women who have sex with women in sub-Saharan Africa, 50–80% of women reported ever having had sexual contact with a man; one in five women had had sex with a man in the preceding year. Among 280 women who have sex with women in Kenya, 7.5% reported to be living with HIV (9.4% of the women who reported having been tested for HIV). Among these women, having had a sexually transmitted infection and having had any male sexual male partner was also associated with HIV infection (Zaidi et al., 2016). Unexpected rates of HIV among lesbian and bisexual women have been attributed to unsafe transactional sex with men generally as well as alarming levels of rape and sexual violence among women and lesbian women, particularly in South Africa (Polders & Wells, 2004), as well as *corrective rape*, in which women are raped because of their perceived sexual orientation or gender identity, motivated by the perpetrator to turn the person heterosexual or to enforce conformity with gender stereotypes (Logie et al., 2020). Matebeni et al. (2013) interviewed 24 self-identifying African lesbians living with HIV in Southern Africa. While battling with their own perceptions of invulnerability and accepting their HIV-positive status, these women had to deal with wide ranging stigmatization, discrimination and misconceptions about risk.

1.10 This Volume

This volume brings together contributions on male same-sex sexuality and HIV from a diversity of disciplinary perspectives. The diversity of contributions illustrates how over the past two decades, the field has rapidly evolved. While before the turn of the century scholarly research on male same-sex sexuality in sub-Saharan Africa was practically non-existent, and awareness that HIV was also disproportionally affecting men who have sex with men in Africa has generated an outbreak of research. Most early studies were of an epidemiological nature, mapping sexual risk behaviours and documenting the HIV prevalence. Other research provided additional insights in the interpersonal, social and cultural contexts of male same-sex sexual expression and HIV or looked at health and legal policy.

Research among men who have sex with men in sub-Saharan Africa is most often conducted in collaboration with the communities that are being studied, albeit to varying degrees. This occurs for practical reasons: firstly, because the behaviour being studied is highly stigmatised and in many African countries illegal; and secondly, because collaboration with communities is essential for gaining access and trust. There is also a growing awareness that partnership with local communities will advance the causes of these communities and is needed if research is to have impact. Such collaborations offer not only opportunities but also challenges (Molyneux et al., 2016; Onyango-Ouma et al., 2009). Best-practice guidelines have been developed to ensure that in the process, the safety and rights of communities are protected (see, for example, The GMT Initiative, 2015). These guidelines played a major role in the development and implementation of the HIV Prevention Trials Network 075 study, a multinational project to assess the feasibility of recruitment and retention of men who have sex with men in sub-Saharan Africa (Sandfort et al., 2020). In their chapter in this book, *Conducting HIV Research with Sexual and Gender Minorities in sub-Saharan Africa: Experiences from Malawi*, Daniel Gondwe and colleagues describe the implementation of the research in Blantyre, Malawi, one of the project's four study sites, and how they dealt with challenges related to recruitment, retention, stakeholder engagement, and mitigation of social harms. Same-sex behaviour is a criminal offence in Malawi. As a result, various strategies had to be used to convince a diverse group of stakeholders about the relevance of the project from the perspective that the Malawi HIV epidemic was a public health and human rights issue, superseding personal and political agendas. Community stakeholders were also engaged in solving problems encountered during study implementation. The various partnerships built during this project advanced HIV prevention, bolstered recruitment and retention, and minimised the risk of social harm to study participants and staff.

Substance use, and alcohol use in particular, have been intensively studied among men who have sex with men in sub-Saharan Africa. Much of this research has assessed actual use but sheds little light on the context in which drinking occurs (Sandfort et al., 2017). In "*Heavy Drinking*" *and HIV Vulnerability among African Male Sex Workers: Narratives from a Community-Based Participatory Study in Nairobi, Kenya*, Robert Lorway and colleagues explore how international health discourse has shaped the meanings, experiences, and subjectivities of male sex workers in Kenya with respect to heavy drinking. Such discourse compels male sex workers to reflect on and enact ways to improve community health, while constructing their sexual health as continually in jeopardy. Accordingly, men reduce getting drunk, locally referred to in Kiswahili as *kulewa*, to the effects of 'poor' individual decision making. Listening to the men's stories, it becomes clear that heavy drinking is much more than this, being a coping response to multiple overlapping forms of oppression faced by men themselves and the wider community of male sex workers.

Two contributions to this volume focus on the prevention and care for men who have sex with men. Formally, attention to HIV prevention for men who have sex with men is increasing in sub-Saharan Africa. A comparison of national strategic plans for the first and the second decade of the twenty-first century shows that an increasing number of countries recognise men who have sex with men as a key population in need of focused HIV prevention and surveillance (Makofane et al., 2013; WHO, 2018). Tara McKay describes in *Struggles for Inclusion; Incorporating Same-Sex Practising Men into National HIV Prevention and Surveillance in African Countries, 2000–2020* how these changes have come about. She draws on a rich collection of archival, qualitative interview and quantitative data. In her contribution, McKay examines whether and when African countries have integrated same-sex practising men into the national HIV responses. She identifies key drivers of inclusion and resistance to inclusion within these responses.

In *Hardship, Public Health, Heshima, Lube and Problem Trees: Forces Shaping Grassroots Organizing Against HIV among Same-Sex Attracted Men in Dar Es Salaam*, Kåre Moen and colleagues describe actions on the ground. They identify various factors influencing the emergence and expansion of grassroots organizing for HIV prevention among same-sex attracted men in Dar es Salaam, Tanzania. Their account is informed by ethnographic fieldwork, including long-term participant observation in community-based groups and interviews with grassroots activists, community members, health care workers, community leaders, policy makers and planners involved in programming focused on same-sex attracted men. The chapter discusses how in the context of hardship, grassroot organizers have organized HIV prevention and care activities, articulating the role of funding agencies as well as local understandings of *heshima*, a concept implying dignity, honour, courtesy and respect, as central to this response. Drawing on the values inherent in heshima, grassroot organisers have found allies in unexpected places, such as the church, and practised reasoned subversion, for instance by establishing alternative sexual lubricant supply lines and, through dialogical education, created widespread community awareness and action.

As described by writers such as Angotti et al. (2019), growing attention to male same-sex sexuality in national HIV policies and the related increased visibility of gay and bisexual men have also triggered a counterproductive response. Similar tendencies are described by Akua O. Gyamerah in her chapter, *Moral Panic and Other Unintended Consequences in Ghana's Paradigm Shift to Address HIV among Men Who Have Sex with Men.* This analyses how in 2011, Ghana came to include men who have sex with men in its national HIV response. It also shows how the criminalisation and stigmatization of male same-sex sexual activities came to shape HIV prevention and care activities, leading to the politicisation of homosexuality in Ghana. This exerted a negative influence on efforts to develop and implement HIV policies and programs for members of this population. When programmes addressing the need of men who have sex with men had to go underground temporarily, men themselves became fearful of accessing HIV services. In response to these developments, important steps have been taken to address the stigma and rights abuse experienced by men who have sex with men and frontline workers.

Together, the contributions in this book encompass something of the diverse scholarship on same-sex sexuality and HIV in sub-Saharan Africa, that has rapidly developed over the past two decennia. This writing, involving African as well as international researchers, has been a major catalyst in the development of policies focused on ending the HIV epidemic among men who have sex with men in a context where for long time little knowledge existed. Not all developments have been even or progressive and there are still major concerns to address, including tackling the criminalisation and stigmatisation of same-sex sexuality and sexual relationships. The hope, however, is that further research will be conducted in such a way, and in partnership with local communities, that it promotes the future health and well-being of all same-sex practising men in sub-Saharan Africa.

References

Adebajo, S., Obianwu, O., Eluwa, G., Vu, L., Oginni, A., Tun, W., Sheehy, M., Ahonsi, B., Bashorun, A., Idogho, O., & Karlyn, A. (2014). Comparison of audio computer assisted self-interview and face-to-face interview methods in eliciting HIV-related risks among men who have sex with men and men who inject drugs in Nigeria. *PLoS One, 9*(1), e81981.

Agardh, C., Weije, F., Agardh, A., Nyoni, J., Ross, M. W., Kashiha, J., & Larsson, M. (2017). Using pharmacists and drugstore workers as sexual healthcare givers: A qualitative study of men who have sex with men in Dar es Salaam, Tanzania. *Global Health Action, 10*(1), 1389181.

Alcala-Alezones, C., Sandfort, T. G. M., Serafino, S., & Reddy, V. (2018). South African men who have sex with both men and women and how they differ from men who have sex with men exclusively. *Journal of Sex Research, 55*(8), 1048–1055.

Anderson, I. W. (1983). Immunological abnormalities in South African homosexual men. *South African Medical Journal, 64*(4), 119–122.

Angotti, N., McKay, T., & Robinson, R. S. (2019). Lgbt visibility and anti-gay backlash. *Sociology of Development, 5*(1), 71–90.

Awondo, P., Geschiere, P., & Reid, G. (2012). Homophobic Africa? Toward a more nuanced view. *African Studies Review, 53*, 145–168.

Babalola, T. K., & Moodley, I. (2020). Assessing the efficiency of health-care facilities in sub-Saharan Africa: A systematic review. *Health Services Research and Managerial Epidemiology, 7*, 2333392820919604.

Balogun, A., Bissell, P., & Saddiq, M. (2020). Negotiating access to the Nigerian healthcare system: The experiences of HIV-positive men who have sex with men. *Culture, Health and Sexuality, 22*(2), 233–246.

Baral, S., Trapence, G., Motimedi, F., Umar, E., Iipinge, S., Dausab, F., & Beyrer, C. (2009). HIV prevalence, risks for HIV infection, and human rights among men who have sex with men (MSM) in Malawi, Namibia, and Botswana. *PLoS One, 4*(3), e4997.

Beyrer, C., Trapence, G., Motimedi, F., Umar, E., Iipinge, S., Dausab, F., & Baral, S. (2010). Bisexual concurrency, bisexual partnerships, and HIV among Southern African men who have sex with men. *Sexually Transmitted Infections, 86*(4), 323–327.

Beyrer, C., Baral, S. D., Van Griensven, F., Goodreau, S. M., Chariyalertsak, S., Wirtz, A. L., & Brookmeyer, R. (2012). Global epidemiology of HIV infection in men who have sex with men. *The Lancet, 380*(9839), 367–377.

Cloete, A., Sanger, N., & Simbayi, L. C. (2011). Are HIV positive women who have sex with women (WSW) an unrecognized and neglected HIV risk group in South Africa? *Journal of AIDS and HIV Research, 3*(1), 1–5.

Cloete, A., Wabiri, N., Simbayi, L., Van der Merwe, L. A., Skinner, D., & Naidoo, D. (2019, July 29–31). *Preliminary results of the first HIV prevalence survey conducted amongst transgender women (TGW) in Southern Africa.* Paper presented at AIDSImpact, London.

Cortés, A. J. (2018). On how role versatility boosts an STI. *Journal of Theoretical Biology, 440*, 66–69.

Couderc, C., Dembele Keita, B., Anoma, C., Wade, A. S., Coulibaly, A., Ehouman, S., Diop, A. K., Yomb, Y., Henry, E., Spire, B., & Laurent, C. (2017). Is PrEP needed for MSM in West Africa? HIV incidence in a prospective multicountry cohort. *Journal of Acquired Immune Deficiency Syndromes, 75*(3), e80–e82.

Coulaud, P. j., Sagaon-Teyssier, L., M'madi Mrenda, B., Maradan, G., Mora, M., Bourrelly, M., Dembélé Keita, B., Keita, A. A., Anoma, C., & Babo Yoro, S. A. (2018). Interest in HIV pre-exposure prophylaxis in men who have sex with men in West Africa (Coh MSM ANRS 12324–Expertise France). *Tropical Medicine and International Health, 23*(10), 1084–1091.

Coulaud, P. J., Sagaon-Teyssier, L., Mimi, M., M'Madi Mrenda, B., Maradan, G., Mora, M., Bourrelly, M., Keita, B. D., Keita, A. A., Anoma, C., Babo Yoro, S. A., Dah, T. T. E., Coulibaly, C., Mensah, E., Agbomadji, S., Bernier, A., Couderc, C., Laurent, C., Spire, B., & Coh, M. S. M. S. G. (2020). Combined sexual behavioral profiles in HIV-seronegative men who have sex with men in West Africa (CohMSM ANRS 12324-Expertise France). *Archives of Sexual Behavior, 49*(1), 331–345.

Cover, R. I. (2018). The proliferation of gender and sexual identities, categories and labels among young people: Emergent taxonomies. In P. Aggleton, R. Cover, D. Leahy, D. Marshall, & M. L. Rasmussen (Eds.), *Youth, sexuality and sexual citizenship* (pp. 278–290). Routledge.

Cover, R. (2020). Populist contestations: Cultural change and the competing languages of sexual and gender identity. *Sexualities*. Advance online publication.

Diamond, L. M. (2004). Emerging perspectives on distinctions between romantic love and sexual desire. *Current Directions in Psychological Science, 13*(3), 116–119.

Duncan, D. T., Park, S. H., Schneider, J. A., Al-Ajlouni, Y. A., Goedel, W. C., Elbel, B., Morganstein, J. G., Ransome, Y., & Mayer, K. H. (2017). Financial hardship, condomless anal intercourse and HIV risk among men who have sex with men. *AIDS and Behavior, 21*(12), 3478–3485.

Eluwa, G. I., Adebajo, S. B., Eluwa, T., Ogbanufe, O., Ilesanmi, O., & Nzelu, C. (2019). Rising HIV prevalence among men who have sex with men in Nigeria: A trend analysis. *BMC Public Health, 19*(1), 1–10.

Epprecht, M. (2006). "Bisexuality" and the politics of normal in African ethnography. *Anthropologica, 48*, 187–201.

Epprecht, M. (2008). *Heterosexual Africa? The history of an idea from the age of exploration to the age of AIDS*. Ohio University Press.

Epprecht, M. (2013). *Hungochani: The history of a dissident sexuality in southern Africa*. McGill-Queen's Press-MQUP.

Essack, Z., Lynch, I., Kaunda, C. J., Stephenson, R., Darbes, L., & van Rooyen, H. (2020). Power relations in sexual agreements among male couples in Southern Africa. *Culture, Health and Sexuality, 22*(8), 904–919.

Fleming, A. F. (1988). Seroepidemiology of human immunodeficiency viruses in Africa. *Biomedicine and Pharmacotherapy, 42*(5), 309–320.

Gyamerah, A. O., Collier, K. L., Reddy, V., & Sandfort, T. G. M. (2019). Sexuality disclosure among Black South African MSM and responses by family. *Journal of Sex Research, 56*(9), 1203–1218.

Hahn, J. A., Woolf-King, S. E., & Muyindike, W. (2011). Adding fuel to the fire: Alcohol's effect on the HIV epidemic in Sub-Saharan Africa. *Current HIV/AIDS Reports, 8*(3), 172–180.

Hessou, P. H. S., Glele-Ahanhanzo, Y., Adekpedjou, R., Ahouada, C., Johnson, R. C., Boko, M., Zomahoun, H. T. V., & Alary, M. (2019). Comparison of the prevalence rates of HIV infection between men who have sex with men (MSM) and men in the general population in sub-Saharan Africa: A systematic review and meta-analysis. *BMC Public Health, 19*(1), 1634.

Howard, B. (2020). *Religion in Africa: Tolerance and trust in leaders are high, but many would allow regulation of religious speech*. Afrobarometer, Dispatch No. 339.

Ireland, P. R. (2013). A macro-level analysis of the scope, causes, and consequences of homophobia in Africa. *African Studies Review, 56*(2), 47–66.

Johnston, L. G., Holman, A., Dahoma, M., Miller, L. A., Kim, E., Mussa, M., Othman, A. A., Kim, A., Kendall, C., & Sabin, K. (2010). HIV risk and the overlap of injecting drug use and high-risk sexual behaviours among men who have sex with men in Zanzibar (Unguja), Tanzania. *International Journal of Drug Policy, 21*(6), 485–492.

Joint United Nations Programme on HIV/AIDS. (2020). *Seizing the moment: Tackling entrenched inequalities to end epidemics*. UNAIDS.

Keshinro, B., Crowell, T. A., Nowak, R. G., Adebajo, S., Peel, S., Gaydos, C. A., Rodriguez-Hart, C., Baral, S. D., Walsh, M. J., Njoku, O. S., Odeyemi, S., Ngo-Ndomb, T., Blattner, W. A., Robb, M. L., Charurat, M. E., Ake, J., & Trust/RV368 Study Group. (2016). High prevalence of HIV, chlamydia and gonorrhoea among men who have sex with men and transgender women attending trusted community centres in Abuja and Lagos, Nigeria. *Journal of the International AIDS Society, 19*(1), 21270.

Kim, H. Y., Grosso, A., Ky-Zerbo, O., Lougue, M., Stahlman, S., Samadoulougou, C., Ouedraogo, G., Kouanda, S., Liestman, B., & Baral, S. (2018). Stigma as a barrier to health care utilization among female sex workers and men who have sex with men in Burkina Faso. *Annals of Epidemiology, 28*(1), 13–19.

Kimani, M., van der Elst, E. M., Chiro, O., Oduor, C., Wahome, E., Kazungu, W., Shally, M., Rinke de Wit, T. F., Graham, S. M., Operario, D., & Sanders, E. J. (2019). PrEP interest and HIV-1 incidence among MSM and transgender women in coastal Kenya. *Journal of the International AIDS Society, 22*(6), e25323.

Kimani, M., van der Elst, E. M., Chirro, O., Wahome, E., Ibrahim, F., Mukuria, N., de Wit, T. F. R., Graham, S. M., Operario, D., & Sanders, E. J. (2021). "I wish to remain HIV negative": Pre-exposure prophylaxis adherence and persistence in transgender women and men who have sex with men in coastal Kenya. *PLoS One, 16*(1), e0244226.

King, R., Barker, J., Nakayiwa, S., Katuntu, D., Lubwama, G., Bagenda, D., Lane, T., Opio, A., & Hladik, W. (2013). Men at risk; a qualitative study on HIV risk, gender identity and violence among men who have sex with men who report high risk behavior in Kampala, Uganda. *PLoS One, 8*(12), e82937.

Kounta, C. H., Sagaon-Teyssier, L., Coulaud, P. J., Mora, M., Maradan, G., Bourrelly, M., Keita, A. A., Yoro, S. B., Anoma, C., Coulibaly, C., Dah, E. T. T., Agbomadji, S., Mensah, E., Bernier, A., Couderc, C., Dembele Keita, B., Laurent, C., Spire, B., & Coh, M. S. M. S. G. (2019). Male clients of male sex workers in West Africa: A neglected high-risk population. *PLoS One, 14*(5), e0212245.

Lahuerta, M., Patnaik, P., Ballo, T., Telly, N., Knox, J., Traore, B., Doumbia, S., & Hakim, A. (2018). HIV prevalence and related risk factors in men who have sex with men in Bamako, Mali: Findings from a bio-behavioral survey using respondent-driven sampling. *AIDS and Behavior, 22*(7), 2079–2088.

Lamontagne, E., d'Elbee, M., Ross, M. W., Carroll, A., Plessis, A. D., & Loures, L. (2018). A socioecological measurement of homophobia for all countries and its public health impact. *European Journal of Public Health, 28*(5), 967–972.

Lane, T., Mogale, T., Struthers, H., McIntyre, J., & Kegeles, S. M. (2008). "They see you as a different thing": The experiences of men who have sex with men with healthcare workers in South African township communities. *Sexually Transmitted Infections, 84*(6), 430–433.

Lane, T., Osmand, T., Marr, A., Struthers, H., McIntyre, J. A., & Shade, S. B. (2016). Brief report: High HIV Incidence in a South African community of men who have sex with men: Results from the Mpumalanga Men's Study, 2012–2015. *Journal of Acquired Immune Deficiency Syndromes, 73*(5), 609–611.

Larmarange, J., Wade, A. S., Diop, A. K., Diop, O., Gueye, K., Marra, A., du Lou, A. D., & for, E. G. (2010). Men who have sex with men (MSM) and factors associated with not using a condom at last sexual intercourse with a man and with a woman in Senegal. *PLoS One, 5*(10), e13189.

Leap, W. L. (2004). Language, belonging and (homo) sexual citizenship in Cape Town, South Africa. In T. Boellstorff & W. Leap (Eds.), *Speaking in queer tongues: Globalization and gay language* (pp. 134–162). University of Illinois Press.

Logie, C. H., Perez-Brumer, A., Mothopeng, T., Latif, M., Ranotsi, A., & Baral, S. D. (2020). Conceptualizing LGBT stigma and associated HIV vulnerabilities among LGBT persons in Lesotho. *AIDS and Behavior, 24*(12), 3462–3472.

Lyons, A., Pitts, M., Smith, G., Grierson, J., Smith, A., McNally, S., & Couch, M. (2011). Versatility and HIV vulnerability: Investigating the proportion of Australian gay men having both insertive and receptive anal intercourse. *The Journal of Sexual Medicine, 8*(8), 2164–2171.

Lyons, C. E., Ketende, S., Diouf, D., Drame, F. M., Liestman, B., Coly, K., Ndour, C., Turpin, G., Mboup, S., & Diop, K. (2017). Potential impact of integrated stigma mitigation interventions in improving HIV/AIDS service delivery and uptake for key populations in Senegal. *Journal of Acquired Immune Deficiency Syndromes (1999), 74*(Suppl 1), S52.

Maartens, G., Wood, R., O'Keefe, E., & Byrne, C. (1997). Independent epidemics of heterosexual and homosexual HIV infection in South Africa—Survival differences. *QJM: Monthly Journal of the Association of Physicians, 90*(7), 449–454.

Magesa, D. J., Mtui, L. J., Abdul, M., Kayange, A., Chiduo, R., Leshabari, M. T., Kayombo, E., & Tungaraza, D. (2014). Barriers to men who have sex with men attending HIV related health services in Dar es Salaam, Tanzania. *Tanzanian Journal of Health Research, 16*(2), 118–126.

Maisto, S. A., & Simons, J. S. (2016). Research on the effects of alcohol and sexual arousal on sexual risk in men who have sex with men: Implications for HIV prevention interventions. *AIDS and Behavior, 20*(1), 158–172.

Makofane, K., Gueboguo, C., Lyons, D., & Sandfort, T. G. M. (2013). Men who have sex with men inadequately addressed in African AIDS National Strategic Plans. *Global Public Health, 8*(2), 129–143.

Matebeni, Z., Reddy, V., Sandfort, T. G. M., & Southey-Swartz, I. (2013). "I thought we are safe": Southern African lesbians' experiences of living with HIV. *Culture, Health and Sexuality, 15* (Suppl), 34–47.

Mbeda, C., Ogendo, A., Lando, R., Schnabel, D., Gust, D. A., Guo, X., Akelo, V., Dominguez, K., Panchia, R., Mbilizi, Y., Chen, Y., Chege, W., Sandfort, T., & on behalf of the HPTN Protocol Team. (2020). Healthcare-related stigma among men who have sex with men and transgender women in sub-Saharan Africa participating in HIV Prevention Trials Network (HPTN) 075 study. *Aids Care, 32*(8), 1052–1060.

Mbiti, J. S. (1990). *African religions & philosophy*. Heinemann.

Mbote, D. K., Sandfort, T. G., Waweru, E., & Zapfel, A. (2018). Kenyan religious leaders' views on same-sex sexuality and gender nonconformity: Religious freedom versus constitutional rights. *The Journal of Sex Research, 55*(4–5), 630–641.

Mendos, L. R. (2019). *State-sponsored homophobia*. ILGA.

Micheni, M., Kombo, B. K., Secor, A., Simoni, J. M., Operario, D., van der Elst, E. M., Mugo, P., Kanungi, J., Sanders, E. J., & Graham, S. M. (2017). Health provider views on improving antiretroviral therapy adherence among men who have sex with men in Coastal Kenya. *AIDS Patient Care STDS, 31*(3), 113–121.

Mimiaga, M. J., Hughto, J. M. W., Biello, K. B., Santostefano, C. M., Kuhns, L. M., Reisner, S. L., & Garofalo, R. (2019). Longitudinal analysis of syndemic psychosocial problems predicting HIV risk behavior among a multicity prospective cohort of sexually active young transgender women in the United States. *Journal of Acquired Immune Deficiency Syndrome, 81*(2), 184–192.

Minter, S. (2000). Do transsexuals dream of gay rights? Getting real about transgender inclusion in the gay rights movement. *New York Law School Journal of Human Rights, 17*, 589–621.

Moen, K., Aggleton, P., Leshabari, M. T., & Middelthon, A.-L. (2014). Same-sex practicing men in Tanzania from 1860 to 2010. *Archives of Sexual Behavior, 43*(6), 1065–1082.

Molyneux, S., Sariola, S., Allman, D., Dijkstra, M., Gichuru, E., Graham, S., Kamuya, D., Gakii, G., Kayemba, B., Kombo, B., Maleche, A., Mbwambo, J., Marsh, V., Micheni, M., Mumba, N., Parker, M., Shio, J., Yah, C., van der Elst, E., & Sanders, E. (2016). Public/community engagement in health research with men who have sex with men in sub-Saharan Africa: Challenges and opportunities. *Health Research Policy and Systems, 14*(1), 40.

Muraguri, N., Tun, W., Okal, J., Broz, D., Raymond, H. F., Kellogg, T., Dadabhai, S., Musyoki, H., Sheehy, M., & Kuria, D. (2015). HIV and STI prevalence and risk factors among male sex workers and other men who have sex with men in Nairobi, Kenya. *Journal of Acquired Immune Deficiency Syndromes, 68*(1), 91–96.

Murray, S. O. (2002). *Homosexualities*. University of Chicago Press.

Musinguzi, G., Bastiaens, H., Matovu, J. K., Nuwaha, F., Mujisha, G., Kiguli, J., Arinaitwe, J., Van Geertruyden, J.-P., & Wanyenze, R. K. (2015). Barriers to condom use among high risk men who have sex with men in Uganda: A qualitative study. *PLoS One, 10*(7), e0132297.

Nelson, L. E., Wilton, L., Agyarko-Poku, T., Zhang, N., Aluoch, M., Thach, C. T., Owiredu Hanson, S., & Adu-Sarkodie, Y. (2015). The association of HIV stigma and HIV/STD knowledge with sexual risk behaviors among adolescent and adult men who have sex with men in Ghana, West Africa. *Research in Nursing and Health, 38*(3), 194–206.

Nowak, R. G., Mitchell, A., Crowell, T. A., Liu, H., Ketende, S., Ramadhani, H. O., Ndembi, N., Adebajo, S., Ake, J., & Michael, N. L. (2019). Individual and sexual network predictors of HIV incidence among men who have sex with men in Nigeria. *Journal of Acquired Immune Deficiency Syndromes, 80*(4), 444–453.

Oginni, O. A., Mapayi, B. M., Afolabi, O. T., Ebuenyi, I. D., Akinsulore, A., & Mosaku, K. S. (2019). Association between risky sexual behavior and a psychosocial syndemic among Nigerian men who have sex with men. *Journal of Gay and Lesbian Mental Health, 23*(2), 168–185.

Ogunbajo, A., Kershaw, T., Kushwaha, S., Boakye, F., Wallace-Atiapah, N. D., & Nelson, L. E. (2018). Barriers, motivators, and facilitators to engagement in HIV care among HIV-infected Ghanaian men who have sex with men (MSM). *AIDS and Behavior, 22*(3), 829–839.

Ogunbajo, A., Iwuagwu, S., Williams, R., Biello, K. B., Kahler, C. W., Sandfort, T. G., & Mimiaga, M. J. (2020). Experiences of minority stress among gay, bisexual, and other men who have sex with men (GBMSM) in Nigeria, Africa: The intersection of mental health, substance use, and HIV sexual risk behavior. *Global Public Health*, 1–15. https://doi.org/10.1080/17441692.2020.1834598.

Okafor, C. N., Christodoulou, J., Bantjes, J., Qondela, T., Stewart, J., Shoptaw, S., Tomlinson, M., & Rotherman-Borus, M. J. (2018). Understanding HIV risk behaviors among young men in South Africa: A syndemic approach. *AIDS and Behavior, 22*(12), 3962–3970.

Okal, J., Luchters, S., Geibel, S., Chersich, M. F., Lango, D., & Temmerman, M. (2009). Social context, sexual risk perceptions and stigma: HIV vulnerability among male sex workers in Mombasa, Kenya. *Culture, Health and Sexuality, 11*(8), 811–826.

Okall, D. O., Otieno, F. O., Nyikuri, M., Mills, L. A., Hardnett, F., Odero, S., Turner, K., & Gust, D. A. (2013). Men who have sex with men in Kisumu, Kenya: Support group membership and knowledge of HIV-risk factors. *Culture, Health and Sexuality, 15*(8), 968–980.

Oldenburg, C. E., Perez-Brumer, A. G., Reisner, S. L., & Mimiaga, M. J. (2015). Transactional sex and the HIV epidemic among men who have sex with men (MSM): Results from a systematic review and meta-analysis. *AIDS and Behavior, 19*(12), 2177–2183.

Ondeng'e, K., Mbeda, C., Ogendo, A., Akelo, V., Guo, X., Chege, W., Hamilton, E. L., Lucas, J., & Sandfort, T. G. M. (2018). *Bisexuality among men who have sex with men and transgender women (MSM&TW) in sub-Saharan Africa: Findings from the HPTN 075 study.* Poster presented at the 22nd International AIDS Conference Amsterdam, Netherlands.

Onyango-Ouma, W., Birungi, H., & Geibel, S. (2009). Engaging men who have sex with men in operations research in Kenya. *Culture, Health and Sexuality, 11*(8), 827–839.

Operario, D., & Nemoto, T. (2010). HIV in transgender communities: Syndemic dynamics and a need for multicomponent interventions. *Journal of Acquired Immune Deficiency Syndromes, 55* (Suppl 2), S91–S93.

Palumbo, P. J., Zhang, Y., Clarke, W., Breaud, A., Sivay, M., Cummings, V., Hamilton, E. L., Guo, X., Ogendo, A., Kayange, N., Panchia, R., Dominguez, K., Chen, Y. Q., Sandfort, T. G. M., & Eshleman, S. H. (2021). Uptake of antiretroviral treatment and viral suppression among men who have sex with men and transgender women in sub-Saharan Africa in an observational cohort study: HPTN 075. *International Journal of Infectious Diseases, 104*, 465–470.

Polders, L., & Wells, H. (2004). *Levels of empowerment among lesbian, gay, bisexual and transgender [LGBT] people in Gauteng, South Africa*. OUT LGBT Wellbeing.

Porter, M. A. (1995). Talking at the margins: Kenyan discourses on homosexuality. In W. Leap (Ed.), *In beyond the lavender lexicon: Authenticity, imagination, and appropriation in lesbian and gay languages* (pp. 133–153). Gordon & Breach.

Poteat, T., Logie, C., Adams, D., Lebona, J., Letsie, P., Beyrer, C., & Baral, S. (2014). Sexual practices, identities and health among women who have sex with women in Lesotho—A mixed-methods study. *Culture, Health and Sexuality, 16*(2), 120–135.

Poteat, T., German, D., & Flynn, C. (2016a). The conflation of gender and sex: Gaps and opportunities in HIV data among transgender women and MSM. *Global Public Health, 11* (7–8), 835–848.

Poteat, T., Scheim, A., Xavier, J., Reisner, S., & Baral, S. (2016b). Global epidemiology of HIV infection and related syndemics affecting transgender people. *Journal of Acquired Immune Deficiency Syndromes, 72*, S210–S219.

Poteat, T., Ackerman, B., Diouf, D., Ceesay, N., Mothopeng, T., Odette, K. Z., Kouanda, S., Ouedraogo, H. G., Simplice, A., Kouame, A., Mnisi, Z., Trapence, G., van der Merwe, L. L. A., Jumbe, V., & Baral, S. (2017). HIV prevalence and behavioral and psychosocial factors among transgender women and cisgender men who have sex with men in 8 African countries: A cross-sectional analysis. *PLoS Medicine, 14*(11), e1002422.

Poushter, J., & Kent, N. (2020). *The global divide on homosexuality persists*. Pew Research Center.

Price, M. A., Rida, W., Mwangome, M., Mutua, G., Middelkoop, K., Roux, S., Okuku, H. S., Bekker, L. G., Anzala, O., Ngugi, E., Stevens, G., Chetty, P., Amornkul, P. N., & Sanders, E. J. (2012). Identifying at-risk populations in Kenya and South Africa: HIV incidence in cohorts of men who report sex with men, sex workers, and youth. *Journal of Acquired Immune Deficiency Syndromes, 59*(2), 185–193.

Quilter, L. A. S., Obondi, E., Kunzweiler, C., Okall, D., Bailey, R. C., Djomand, G., Otieno-Nyunya, B., Otieno, F., & Graham, S. M. (2019). Prevalence and correlates of and a risk score to identify asymptomatic anorectal gonorrhoea and chlamydia infection among men who have sex with men in Kisumu, Kenya. *Sexually Transmitted Infections, 95*(3), 201–211.

Ras, G., Simson, I., Anderson, R., Prozesky, O., & Hamersma, T. (1983). Acquired immunodeficiency syndrome. A report of 2 South African cases. *South African Medical Journal, 64*(4), 140–142.

Rebe, K., Hoosen, N., & McIntyre, J. A. (2019). Strategies to improve access for MSM in low-income and middle-income countries. *Current Opinion in HIV and AIDS, 14*(5), 387–392.

Rispel, L. C., Metcalf, C. A., Cloete, A., Reddy, V., & Lombard, C. (2011). HIV prevalence and risk practices among men who have sex with men in two South African cities. *Journal of Acquired Immune Deficiency Syndromes, 57*(1), 69–76.

Sanders, E. J., Graham, S. M., Okuku, H. S., van der Elst, E. M., Muhaari, A., Davies, A., Peshu, N., Price, M., McClelland, R. S., & Smith, A. D. (2007). HIV-1 infection in high risk men who have sex with men in Mombasa, Kenya. *Aids, 21*(18), 2513–2520.

Sanders, E. J., Okuku, H. S., Smith, A. D., Mwangome, M., Wahome, E., Fegan, G., Peshu, N., Van Der Elst, E. M., Price, M. A., & McClelland, R. S. (2013). High HIV-1 incidence, correlates of HIV-1 acquisition, and high viral loads following seroconversion among men who have sex with men in Coastal Kenya. *Aids, 27*(3), 437–446.

Sandfort, T. G. M., Baumann, L. R., Matebeni, Z., Reddy, V., & Southey-Swartz, I. (2013a). Forced sexual experiences as risk factor for self-reported HIV infection among southern African lesbian and bisexual women. *PLoS One, 8*(1), e53552.

Sandfort, T. G. M., Yi, H., Knox, J., & Reddy, V. (2013b). Sexual partnership types as determinant of HIV risk in South African MSM: An event-level cluster analysis. *AIDS and Behavior, 17*(1), 23–32.

Sandfort, T. G. M., Lane, T., Dolezal, C., & Reddy, V. (2015). Gender expression and risk of HIV infection among black South African men who have sex with men. *AIDS and Behavior, 19*(12), 2270–2279.

Sandfort, T. G. M., Knox, J. R., Alcala, C., El-Bassel, N., Kuo, I., & Smith, L. R. (2017). Substance use and HIV risk among men who have sex with men in Africa: A systematic review. *Journal of Acquired Immune Deficiency Syndromes, 76*(2), e34.

Sandfort, T. G. M., Bos, H., & Reddy, V. (2018). Gender expression and mental health in Black South African men who have sex with men: Further explorations of unexpected findings. *Archives of Sexual Behavior, 47*, 2481–2490.

Sandfort, T. G. M., Dominguez, K., Kayange, N., Ogendo, A., Panchia, R., Chen, Y. Q., Chege, W., Cummings, V., Guo, X., Hamilton, E. L., Stirratt, M., & Eshleman, S. H. (2019). HIV testing and the HIV care continuum among sub-Saharan African men who have sex with men and transgender women screened for participation in HPTN 075. *PLoS One, 14*(5), e0217501.

Sandfort, T. G. M., Hamilton, E. L., Marais, A., Guo, X., Sugarman, J., Chen, Y. Q., Cummings, V., Dadabhai, S., Dominguez, K., Panchia, R., Schnabel, D., Zulu, F., Reynolds, D., Radebe, O., Mbeda, C., Kamba, D., Kanyemba, B., Ogendo, A., Stirratt, M., Chege, W., Lucas, J., Fawzy, M., McKinstry, L. A., & Eshleman, S. H. (2020). The feasibility of recruiting and retaining men who have sex with men and transgender women in a multinational prospective HIV prevention research cohort study in sub-Saharan Africa (HPTN 075). *Journal of the International AIDS Society, 23*, e25600.

Sandfort, T. G. M., Mbilizi, Y., Sanders, E. J., Guo, X., Cummings, V., Hamilton, E. L., Akelo, V., Panchia, R., Dominguez, K., Stirratt, M. J., Chege, W., Lucas, J., Gaydos, C. A., Chen, Y. Q., & Eshleman, S. H. (2021). HIV incidence in a multinational cohort of men and transgender women who have sex with men in sub-Saharan Africa: Findings from HPTN 075. *PLoS One, 16*(2), e0247195.

Selvam, S. G., & Collicutt, J. (2013). The ubiquity of the character strengths in African traditional religion: A thematic analysis. In H. Knoop & A. Fave (Eds.), *Well-being and cultures* (pp. 83–102). Springer.

Sevelius, J. M., Keatley, J., Calma, N., & Arnold, E. (2016). “I am not a man”: Trans-specific barriers and facilitators to PrEP acceptability among transgender women. *Global Public Health, 11*(7-8), 1060–1075.

Sheehy, M., Tun, W., Vu, L., Adebajo, S., Obianwu, O., & Karlyn, A. (2014). High levels of bisexual behavior and factors associated with bisexual behavior among men having sex with men (MSM) in Nigeria. *Aids Care, 26*(1), 116–122.

Smith, A., Kimani, J., Kabuti, R., Weatherburn, P., Fearon, E., & Bourne, A. (2021). HIV burden and correlates of infection among transfeminine persons and cisgender men who have sex with men in Nairobi: An observational study. *The Lancet HIV*. https://doi.org/10.1016/S2352-3018(20)30310-6.

Stahlman, S., Liestman, B., Ketende, S., Kouanda, S., Ky-Zerbo, O., Lougue, M., Diouf, D., Anato, S., Tchalla, J., Bamba, A., Drame, F. M., Ezouatchi, R., Kouame, A., & Baral, S. D. (2016). Characterizing the HIV risks and potential pathways to HIV infection among transgender women in Cote d’Ivoire, Togo and Burkina Faso. *Journal of the International AIDS Society, 19*, 5–16.

Stankov, L., & Lee, J. (2016). Nastiness, morality and religiosity in 33 nations. *Personality and Individual Differences, 99*, 56–66.

Stannah, J., Dale, E., Elmes, J., Staunton, R., Beyrer, C., Mitchell, K. M., & Boily, M.-C. (2019). HIV testing and engagement with the HIV treatment cascade among men who have sex with men in Africa: A systematic review and meta-analysis. *The Lancet HIV, 6*(11), e769–e787.

Sullivan, P. S., Phaswana-Mafuya, N., Baral, S. D., Valencia, R., Zahn, R., Dominguez, K., Yah, C. S., Jones, J., Kgatitswe, L. B., McNaghten, A. D., Siegler, A. J., Sanchez, T. H., & Bekker, L. G. (2020). HIV prevalence and incidence in a cohort of South African men and transgender women who have sex with men: The Sibanye Methods for Prevention Packages Programme (MP3) project. *Journal of the International AIDS Society, 23*(Suppl 6), e25591.

Sutherland, C., Roberts, B., Gabriel, N., Struwig, J., & Gordon, S. (2016). *Progressive prudes: A survey of attitudes towards homosexuality & gender non-conformity in South Africa*. The Other Foundation.

Szulc, Ł., & Dhoest, A. (2013). The internet and sexual identity formation: Comparing Internet use before and after coming out. *Communications, 38*(4), 347–365.

Tat, S. A., Marrazzo, J. M., & Graham, S. M. (2015). Women who have sex with women living in low- and middle-income countries: A systematic review of sexual health and risk behaviors. *LGBT Health, 2*(2), 91–104.

The GMT Initiative. (2015). *Respect, protect, fulfil: Best practices guidance in conducting HIV research with gay, bisexual, and other men who have sex with men (MSM) in rights-constrained environments*. amfAR.

Thompson, K. D. (2015). Discreet talk about supernatural sodomy, transgressive gender performance, and male same-sex desire in Zanzibar Town. *GLQ: A Journal of Lesbian and Gay Studies, 21*(4), 521–559.

Trans*Alliance, Nduta, S., Smith, L., & Okeyo, N. (2020). *Transform: A report of the National Transgender Discrimination Survey in Kenya (NTDS)—A baseline study of transgender persons in Kenya: Life experiences and access to health services*. Epilson Publishers.

United Nations Office of Drugs and Crime. (2019). *World drug report 2019*. United Nations.

Valente, P. K., Mantell, J. E., Masvawure, T. B., Tocco, J. U., Restar, A. J., Gichangi, P., Chabeda, S. V., Lafort, Y., & Sandfort, T. G. M. (2020). "I couldn't afford to resist": Condom negotiations between male sex workers and male clients in Mombasa, Kenya. *AIDS and Behavior, 24*(3), 925–937.

Van der Elst, E. M., Smith, A. D., Gichuru, E., Wahome, E., Musyoki, H., Muraguri, N., Fegan, G., Duby, Z., Bekker, L. G., & Bender, B. (2013). Men who have sex with men sensitivity training reduces homoprejudice and increases knowledge among Kenyan healthcare providers in coastal Kenya. *Journal of the International AIDS Society, 16*, 18748.

Wade, A. S., Kane, C. T., Diallo, P. A. N., Diop, A. K., Gueye, K., Mboup, S., Ndoye, I., & Lagarde, E. (2005). HIV infection and sexually transmitted infections among men who have sex with men in Senegal. *Aids, 19*(18), 2133–2140.

Wahome, E. W., Graham, S. M., Thiong'o, A. N., Mohamed, K., Oduor, T., Gichuru, E., Mwambi, J., Prins, P. M., van der Elst, E., & Sanders, P. E. J. (2020). PrEP uptake and adherence in relation to HIV-1 incidence among Kenyan men who have sex with men. *EClinicalMedicine, 26*, 100541.

Wanyenze, R. K., Musinguzi, G., Matovu, J. K., Kiguli, J., Nuwaha, F., Mujisha, G., Musinguzi, J., Arinaitwe, J., & Wagner, G. J. (2016). "If you tell people that you had sex with a fellow man, it is hard to be helped and treated": Barriers and opportunities for increasing access to HIV services among men who have sex with men in Uganda. *PLoS One, 11*(1), e0147714.

Wei, C., & Raymond, H. F. (2011). Preference for and maintenance of anal sex roles among men who have sex with men: Sociodemographic and behavioral correlates. *Archives of Sexual Behavior, 40*(4), 829–834.

WHO. (2014). *Global status report on alcohol and health*. World Health Organization.

WHO. (2018). *Report on key populations in African HIV/AIDS: National strategic plans*. WHO Regional Office for Africa.

Wiley, J. A., & Herschkorn, S. J. (1989). Homosexual role separation and AIDS epidemics: Insights from elementary models. *The Journal of Sex Research, 26*(4), 434–449.

Williamson, C., & Martin, D. P. (2005). Origin, diversity and spread of HIV-1. In S. Abdool Karim & Q. Abdool Karim (Eds.), *HIV/AIDS in South Africa* (pp. 109–118). Cambridge University Press.

Wirtz, A. L., Kamba, D., Jumbe, V., Trapence, G., Gubin, R., Umar, E., Strömdahl, S. K., Beyrer, C., & Baral, S. D. (2014). A qualitative assessment of health seeking practices among and provision practices for men who have sex with men in Malawi. *BMC International Health and Human Rights, 14*(1), 1–11.

Wirtz, A. L., Trapence, G., Kamba, D., Gama, V., Chalera, R., Jumbe, V., Kumwenda, R., Mangochi, M., Helleringer, S., & Beyrer, C. (2017). Geographical disparities in HIV prevalence and care among men who have sex with men in Malawi: Results from a multisite cross-sectional survey. *The Lancet HIV, 4*(6), e260–e269.

Woolf-King, S. E., Steinmaus, C. M., Reingold, A. L., & Hahn, J. A. (2013). An update on alcohol use and risk of HIV infection in sub-Saharan Africa: Meta-analysis and future research directions. *The International Journal of Alcohol and Drug Research, 2*(1), 99–110.

Zaidi, S. S., Ocholla, A. M., Otieno, R. A., & Sandfort, T. G. M. (2016). Women who have sex with women in Kenya and their sexual and reproductive health. *LGBT Health, 3*(2), 139–145.

Chapter 2
Conducting HIV Research with Sexual and Gender Minorities in Sub-Saharan Africa: Experiences from Malawi

Daniel K. Gondwe, Brian Minalga, Russell Campbell, Erica L. Hamilton, and Jonathan Paul Lucas

Conducting HIV prevention research with sexual and gender minorities in social and political settings that criminalize same-sex behaviour poses numerous challenges including recruitment, retention, stakeholder engagement and social harms mitigation. Research staff are responsible for assessing these challenges and developing appropriate responses prior to study implementation. The Malawi College of Medicine-Johns Hopkins University Research Project participated in HPTN 075, to assess the feasibility of recruitment and retention of men who have sex with men in sub-Saharan Africa. Considering the logistical and ethical challenges of conducting the study in Malawi, where the legal system considers same-sex behaviour a criminal offence, the study team utilized a palette of engagement methods to implement this study safely and successfully. Stakeholders were persuaded about the study importance from the perspective that the Malawi HIV epidemic is a public health and human rights issue that supersedes personal and political agendas. Unique recruitment and retention methods resulted in 100 participants being safely enrolled within 18 weeks with an 86% retention rate at 52 weeks. While the study was designed for cisgender men who have sex with men, 27 transgender women were also enrolled. Engaging community stakeholders in problem solving to study challenges is critical for the development of shared responsibility for HIV prevention research. In countries where same-sex behaviour is criminalized, partnership

D. K. Gondwe (✉)
Malawi College of Medicine – Johns Hopkins University Research Project, Blantyre, Malawi
e-mail: dgondwe@jhu.medcol.mw

B. Minalga · R. Campbell
Office of HIV/AIDS Network Coordination, Fred Hutchinson Cancer Research Center, Seattle, WA, USA
e-mail: bminalga@fredhutch.org; rcampbel@fredhutch.org

E. L. Hamilton · J. P. Lucas
FHI 360, Durham, NC, USA
e-mail: EHamilton@fhi360.org; JLucas@fhi360.org

T. Sandfort (ed.), *Male Same-sex Sexuality and HIV in Sub-Saharan Africa*, Social Aspects of HIV 7, https://doi.org/10.1007/978-3-030-73726-9_2

building can advance HIV prevention, bolster recruitment and retention, and minimize risk of social harm to study participants and staff.

2.1 Introduction

This chapter shares lessons learned from a HIV-related study designed to assess the feasibility of recruitment and retention of cisgender men who have sex with men in sub-Saharan Africa. Findings could prove beneficial to organizations engaging cisgender men who have sex with men and transgender women in countries that criminalize same-sex behaviour. The chapter focuses on the engagement strategies utilized by the College of Medicine-Johns Hopkins Research Project in Malawi, one of four clinical research sites participating in a larger study.

2.2 Criminalization of Homosexuality and the HIV Epidemic in Malawi

Malawi is one of 38 countries in Africa that criminalizes homosexuality (Amnesty International, 2013). Men who have sex with men and transgender people can be prosecuted under Malawi's Penal Code, which criminalizes consensual same-sex sexual activity (Commonwealth Lawyers Association, 2015). Section 153 of the Penal Code criminalizes anyone who has intercourse with someone of the same sex. This is punishable by 14 years in prison. Section 154 criminalizes anyone who *attempts* to have intercourse with someone of the same sex. This is punishable by up to 7 years in prison. Section 156 and Section 137A criminalizes "indecent practices" between two men and between two women. Both of these offences are punishable by up to 5 years in prison.

In Malawi, men who have sex with men and transgender women frequently participate in sex work and are thus subject to sections of the Penal Code that target sex workers as well (Commonwealth Lawyers Association, 2015). Sections 180 (d) and (e) punish anyone who commits any indecent act publicly. These offences are considered misdemeanours. The first offence is subject to imprisonment for up to 6 months, and each subsequent offence for up to 18 months.

Anti-homosexuality laws create barriers to HIV prevention and treatment services for marginalized populations (Fay et al., 2011). Men who have sex with men and transgender women are more likely to experience discrimination when accessing health services and are less likely, compared to heterosexual individuals, to seek medical services, including HIV prevention and treatment (UNAIDS, 2016). As a result, many men who have sex with men and transgender women who are vulnerable to HIV and other sexually transmitted infections (STIs) may fear accessing crucial treatment for HIV and other medical issues (Ayala & Santos, 2016). This may lead to a late diagnosis of HIV, which can be costly and difficult to treat (Ayala & Santos, 2016). The stigma and violence experienced by men who have sex with men and transgender women in Malawi as a result of these laws are in part responsible for difficulties in accessing HIV testing, prevention and treatment services and disclosure of HIV status (Fay et al., 2011). This social and structural discrimination against sexual and gender minorities has been shown to impact HIV incidence in the country (UNAIDS, 2017).

In 2016, Malawi had approximately 36,000 new HIV cases and approximately 24,000 AIDS-related deaths. An estimated 1,000,000 people were living with HIV in 2016, among whom 66% were accessing antiretroviral therapy. Among people living with HIV, approximately 59% had suppressed viral loads.

Men who have sex with men have been identified as a key affected population in Malawi, accounting for 17.3% of people living with HIV in the country (UNAIDS, 2017). An estimated one in five men who have sex with men is living with HIV, a prevalence that is two times that of heterosexual men in Malawi. Results from a cross-sectional survey conducted by Wirtz et al. (2017) found that in seven of the 28 districts surveyed 30–45% of men who have sex with men did not know their HIV status. Among these men, it was common to have multiple sex partners and exchange sex for commodities. This survey also found that 39% of men who have sex with men had experienced some form of human rights abuse.

2.3 A Research Project for Men Who Have Sex with Men in Malawi

Recognizing the importance of HIV prevention research for cisgender men who have sex with men, the Malawi College of Medicine-Johns Hopkins University Research Project (the Project), based in Blantyre, Malawi, began to seek out research opportunities inclusive of this marginalized population. Participation in the HPTN 075 study conducted by the HIV Prevention Trials Network (HPTN) proved to be one such opportunity. HPTN is a worldwide clinical trials network that brings together investigators, ethicists and community and other partners to develop and test the safety and efficacy of interventions to prevent the acquisition and transmission of HIV (HIV Prevention Trials Network, 2018). Studies conducted by the network evaluate new HIV prevention interventions and strategies in populations and geographical regions that bear a disproportionate burden of infection.

The study was a multi-country prospective cohort study that sought to determine the feasibility of recruiting and retaining cisgender men who have sex with men in preparation for future large-scale HIV prevention activities in sub-Saharan Africa (HIV Prevention Trials Network 075, 2018; Sandfort et al., 2020). Transgender women were not excluded from participating in the study, although they were not specifically named as a population for recruitment, and their enrolment was unexpected. The larger study was conducted at four clinical research sites (one each in

Kenya and Malawi, and two in South Africa) and sought to enrol 400 participants aged 18–44 years who reported having had anal sex with a man in the previous 3 months. Each site enrolled approximately 100 participants and followed each participant for 12 months. Five study visits were conducted with each participant. They involved structured HIV behavioural assessments, medical examinations, and the collection of biological samples.

In Malawi, the study was conducted by the College of Medicine-Johns Hopkins Research Project, which was established in 1989 and housed within Queen Elizabeth Central Hospital, a public hospital located in the centre of Blantyre. The Project involves research collaborations with four HIV Clinical Research Networks of the US National Institutes of Health to prevent, treat and manage HIV and AIDS in adults, couples and children. Given their expertise in the conduct of HIV prevention and treatment research and their understanding of the HIV prevention needs of cisgender men who have sex with men, researchers involved in the Project had a keen interest in the study.

2.4 Developing a Risk Mitigation Plan

Given stigma, discrimination and criminalization of homosexuality in Malawi, innovative community involvement approaches were needed to protect participants and staff from violence and/or imprisonment. This was the first time the College of Medicine-Johns Hopkins Research Project had ever recruited cisgender men who have sex with men for study participation. The team identified the need to proactively address concerns related to potential social harms, strengthen community rapport and plan for community engagement. The team's approach was based on published *Good Participatory Practice Guidelines* (AVAC & UNAIDS, 2011) and the *Guidelines to Respect, Protect and Fulfill the Needs of Men Who Have Sex with Men in HIV Research* (amfAR et al., 2015). These documents helped conceptualize and develop a comprehensive risk mitigation plan.

The Good Participatory Practice Guidelines from the AIDS Vaccine Advocacy Coalition (AVAC) and the Joint United Nations Programme on HIV/AIDS (UNAIDS) (2011) outline effective community engagement strategies for designing and conducting biomedical HIV prevention research and reflect a set of values—respect, mutual understanding, integrity, transparency, autonomy and accountability—that provide the foundation for positive, collaborative and mutually beneficial relationships that trial funders, sponsors, and implementers can foster with all other stakeholders. The Guidelines to Respect, Protect and Fulfill the Needs of Men Who Have Sex with Men in HIV Research provide recommendations to establish mutually beneficial partnerships between researchers and community-based organizations during research conceptualization, implementation and dissemination (amfAR et al., 2015). The guidelines focus specifically on protecting the rights and safety of men who have sex with men in low- and middle-income countries.

The study protocol team required risk mitigation plans be developed by all of the participating study sites, to ensure study implementation complied with the community engagement guidelines provided by AVAC and amfAR. The purpose of these plans was to protect the cisgender men who have sex with men community by identifying and assessing potential safety risks for participants and clinical research staff. To identify these risks in Malawi, research staff worked closely with a local community-based organization known as the Center for Development of People (CEDEP). The research team also established rapport and gained support from the broader community, including health authorities, media, tribal and religious leaders, the local police and the Project's Community Advisory Board. These community stakeholders provided guidance on potential risks the research team might encounter during the conduct of the study. Notable risks included insensitive treatment by study staff and disclosure of sexual orientation, legal repercussions from study participation, and negative media coverage of the study population or study staff. Once potential risks had been identified by the key stakeholders, they worked with research staff to develop culturally appropriate risk mitigation procedures. Two committees were formed to carry out the risk mitigation plan: a protocol advisory committee and an emergency committee.

2.5 Addressing the Concerns of Study Staff

The HPTN solicited applications from several sites in sub-Saharan Africa for study participation. When the Malawi site received the invitation, two researchers at the site discussed their interest in conducting a study that would enrol men who had sex with other men, with other clinic staff. Many were hesitant to take on the study due to individual stigma, religious beliefs and the threat of being criminalized under the part of the Malawi penal code that punishes the providers of services to men who have sex with men or transgender women (Commonwealth Lawyers Association, 2015). As one provider argued:

> What would happen if I consented someone for this study, I signed their consent form, and they dropped the consent form at the market? If someone finds that consent form and sees my name on it, I may be imprisoned.

The two researchers at the Project advocated strongly for the importance of working with cisgender men who have sex with men and transgender women from a public health perspective, as Malawian sexual and gender minorities often have sex with both men and women to satisfy not only their individual needs but also the social and cultural expectation to marry and have children. This situation, they argued, increases not only the vulnerability of cisgender men who have sex with men and transgender women to HIV, but also the vulnerability of their female sex partners. Understanding the need to provide care to cisgender men who have sex with men, the study staff eventually agreed on the importance of participating in the study. Even after agreeing to conduct the study, however, some clinical staff reported not disclosing their study collaboration to religious leaders and families due to stigma and the fear of being ostracized.

2.6 Developing Meaningful Partnerships with Stakeholders

Engaging community members in problem solving issues that affect them is a fundamental principle of HIV prevention research (AVAC & UNAIDS, 2011). It is a critical strategy for partnership building to advance HIV prevention efforts, particularly with marginalized groups (amfAR et al., 2015). Effective collaboration with influential community stakeholders can aid in the development of shared responsibility and community ownership of HIV prevention research (AVAC & UNAIDS, 2011). As such, this strategy was critical for the Project to garner support for study implementation.

Before initiating the study, the Project sought training and support from the study protocol team to develop plans for risk mitigation, community engagement, recruitment, and retention. The Project also performed a community mapping exercise, with guidance from the study protocol team, to better understand the range of organizations and entities whose engagement would ensure the target population could be safely and effectively enrolled in the study. Those most notable included CEDEP, the site's Community Advisory Board, local law enforcement, media, community gatekeepers and the Institutional Review Board (IRB).

2.6.1 Center for the Development of People (CEDEP)

CEDEP is a community-based organization that provides services to approximately 2450 individuals in Malawi. Its mission is to protect the human rights of marginalized people in Malawi, specifically cisgender men who have sex with men and sex workers. In preparation for the study, the Project began working with CEDEP to gain a better understanding of the needs of cisgender men who have sex with men. Due to the social stigma associated with homosexuality, cisgender men who have sex with men were hesitant to seek medical care for fear of breach of confidentiality and judgement by medical care providers. Many cisgender men who have sex with men had negative experiences when seeking medical care at local hospitals and clinics. As reported by one man:

> I went to the hospital because I had warts in my bottom. The nurse who was treating me brought other nurses in to examine me and they kept asking me why I had warts on my bottom and that the warts should have been in the front. I was so embarrassed. I never returned.

Because the number of cisgender men who have sex with men in Blantyre is relatively small, word spread quickly about such negative experiences, and the community became distrustful of medical providers.

CEDEP trained medical providers from the Project in cultural responsiveness to prepare them to provide client-centred care for cisgender men who have sex with men and transgender women. These sessions covered topics including stigma and discrimination, sexual identity and coming out, anal sex and other common same-sex sexual practices, HIV and STI, condoms and lubricants, sexual risk reduction, and mental health. Once the study staff developed the capacity to provide appropriate care, formal referral mechanisms were established such that CEDEP could refer clients to the Project for the treatment of STIs and other minor medical conditions. This service was provided to any referral from CEDEP and was not reserved only for the people who enrolled in the study. The study staff also developed procedures to ensure study participants' confidentiality. All staff who interacted with participants signed confidentiality agreements and were informed that any disclosure of information about study participants was subject to disciplinary action including termination.

2.6.2 Community Advisory Board

In 2014, the Project initiated discussions about the study with its Community Advisory Board (CAB). The Board had been established in 2003 and had worked with the Project on a multitude of studies. The study team felt strongly about ensuring buy-in from the Board, considering the sensitivity needed to enrol cisgender men who have sex with men. In an environment where members of this population are interpersonally stigmatized and systematically targeted as criminals for their same-sex behaviour, the study team needed a core group of broader community who could help champion and protect the study. The Board played an important role in facilitating stakeholder engagement in the community as the study team built a foundation for the recruitment and retention of this unique study population. Board members included community representatives, a police officer, religious leaders, health care workers, opinion leaders, a staff member from CEDEP and a human rights lawyer with experience defending cisgender men who have sex with men in Malawi charged with same-sex behaviour.

As with other study stakeholders, the CAB expressed several initial concerns about the study. Some Board members cited religious and cultural beliefs that morally positioned them against homosexuality and felt that they could not endorse the study from a personal, moral standpoint. Furthermore, some Board members believed hosting the study in Blantyre might encourage same-sex behaviour in the community by opening discussions about homosexuality and rewarding study participation. They also expressed concern that they might be perceived by the broader community as somehow associated with the gay community if they supported the study, which might harm their personal reputations in the community. Moral opposition to homosexuality was widespread locally, and thus they were concerned that, regardless of their personal beliefs, the broader community would vehemently oppose the study. Board members themselves expressed discomfort talking about same-sex behaviour, and the Board was reluctant to accept the study in these early discussions.

Considering the initial response of the CAB, the study team decided to provide educational training for the Board with support from CEDEP. The training aimed to educate Board members about the communities of cisgender men who have sex with men, provide information about the HIV epidemic among cisgender men who have sex with men, and contextualize the epidemic within the broader Malawian HIV epidemic. During the training, the study team and CEDEP argued for the urgency of responding to the HIV epidemic among cisgender men who have sex with men from a public health perspective, given that many such men in Malawi also have sex with women. When the community viral load among cisgender men who have sex with men is high, trainers explained, HIV proliferates among the general population. Trainers therefore built a central, persuasive argument about public health in Malawi: if cisgender men who have sex with men are affected by HIV, then inevitably, everyone in the community is affected by HIV. The team used this public health lens to shift conversation away from stigma-laden narratives about the study population itself towards the value of conducting HIV research that would benefit everyone. The team further argued that because HIV among cisgender men who have sex with men in Malawi had been severely understudied, the study had the potential to lay the foundation for a public health benefit never before seen in Malawi.

As CAB members participated in the training, their attitudes about the study began to evolve. Board members responded favourably to the public health argument, adding personal sentiments that their sisters, daughters and other female family members might be less vulnerable to HIV if cisgender men who have sex with men had greater HIV prevention support. After seeing objective epidemiological data and discussing the public health implications of HIV among cisgender men who have sex with men as situated within the generalized epidemic, Board members began to develop a sense that the HIV epidemic could not be controlled without including cisgender men who have sex with men in the public health response. A facilitator of the training stated:

> The staff and CAB members were apprehensive about the training at first, but once they began asking questions, you could see that they really wanted to help. But they were afraid because of what they had been taught about homosexuality and how the community would react if they discovered they were conducting a study for men who have sex with men. The training helped them recognize that heterosexuals and homosexuals are all people.

The study team also responded to the Board's moral concerns about the study by invoking the Malawian cultural values of coexistence and helping those in need. The study team noted that while same-sex behaviour had become legally penalized in recent years, religious and cultural traditions have always encouraged Malawians to help those in need. Through the sensitization training and subsequent discussions,

Board members began to see men who have sex with men as populations in need—especially concerning the HIV epidemic. The study team developed a moral imperative argument rooted in a cultural tradition, not legal practice: men who have sex with men have unique needs that must be met, regardless of personal beliefs about same-sex behaviour. Board members began to understand that to ignore the HIV epidemic among vulnerable populations was to dishonour the Malawian tradition of helping those in need. When asked about participation in the sensitization training, one Board representative stated:

> This road was not easy. In our community we do not support man-to-man sexual behavior. But we help people who need help. We cannot end the HIV epidemic in our community if we do not address the HIV epidemic in men who have sex with men. They are a part of our community.

These discussions took place within the context of a broader public discourse in Malawi about homosexuality and human rights. Several highly publicized media reports were released about the same time, documenting human rights abuses in the gay community in Malawi. This broader discourse bolstered the study team's arguments to the CAB regarding the importance of meeting the health and human rights needs of gay Malawians—as well as the value of the study. The research team presented the study as a research opportunity to better address HIV among this understudied population. By the time the clinical research site was ready to begin recruiting participants, the Board not only understood the value of the study but also advocated for it from two main perspectives: (1) gathering information could eventually help improve community health and lower overall HIV incidence and prevalence in Malawi and (2) the study aligned with Malawian cultural values of helping those in need.

2.6.3 Law Enforcement

Obtain buy-in from law enforcement officials prior to the initiation of the study was deemed critically important. This was accomplished through a series of face-to-face meetings in eight communities from the proposed study catchment area. Representatives from the clinical research site along with representatives from CEDEP conducted training on the health and legal needs of cisgender men who have sex with men. It took several weeks to obtain support from law enforcement officials, who, like the CAB, had strong religious views related to homosexuality. One CEDEP representative stated:

> While homosexuality is illegal in Malawi, the law enforcement officials in Malawi agreed to protect cisgender men who have sex with men who were threatened, blackmailed or assaulted. Law enforcement recognized their responsibility to protect all people and gave guidance to the Project on how to conduct the study in the context of the law.

A law enforcement officer who worked with the Project stated:

> While laws against homosexuality exist, they are not enforced generally. It is enforced if you're caught, which means actually seeing the act and having someone to testify that they saw you in the act.

This quote is one example of how law enforcements officials were willing to offer ways to work around the law for the benefit of study participants.

Law enforcement officials also recommended working with community police officers. These officers are placed in communities to help crack down on crime quickly. One of the community police officers was appointed to the CAB and the Protocol Advisory Committee to provide guidance in the event of a study participant or study staff member being arrested.

2.6.4 Media

Years prior to the initiation of the study, the Project had established a solid working relationship with the media. At the time of the study, radio was the main media outlet in Blantyre. In 2003, negative media reports related to cisgender men who have sex with men and transgender women in Malawi had been broadcast. When the clinical research team approached representatives of the media about this negative messaging, media representatives initially were resistant, in alignment with public opinion. However, after receiving cultural responsiveness training from CEDEP, the media outlets in Blantyre ceased publishing these negative reports.

To prevent further negative reports, the clinical research site established a formal media group consisting of approximately 50 news media representatives (two each from 25 outlets). The Project met with the media group every 2 months to discuss media topics related to the research being conducted by the Project and provide them with training around HIV prevention and treatment. In turn, the media began making requests of the Project to speak about homosexuality on the radio. However, site staff opted not to speak on the subject to minimize the risk of stigma and potential violence against participants and the clinical research site staff. Out of safety concerns, the clinical research site opted not to educate the broader community about the study, but their good relationship with the media helped to prepare them in case a public response would be needed.

2.6.5 Community Gatekeepers

As previously mentioned, Malawi is a country known for its conservative views toward same-sex sexual practices. The views of faith and community leaders are widely respected, and those individuals who espouse or support views outside of the religious or community norms are often met with disapproval. Understanding the important role of the various social, political, and religious traditions in Malawi, faith leaders, chiefs, and respected community leaders were engaged prior to the launch of the study. Similar to engagement with the media, clinical research site staff organized three meetings with community gatekeepers to accomplish the following:

- allow gatekeepers to share thoughts on issues related to cisgender men who have sex with men in the community
- discuss health care in general and related to HIV among cisgender men who have sex with men
- provide an overview of the study and solicit their thoughts on the study and issues that might arise from conducting it
- receive permission to engage cisgender men who have sex with men residing in their communities

This engagement strategy proved beneficial. During the meetings, clinical research site staff provided general HIV updates and also introduced the topic of the impact of excluding cisgender men who have sex with men from HIV prevention and treatment strategies. In response, local leaders readily acknowledged that cisgender men who have sex with men are in the community and have always been a part of the community as husbands, fathers, brothers, uncles and cousins, and yet this is not often discussed. Gatekeepers also acknowledged that stigma existed but offered help to the research team discreetly. One chief discouraged publicizing the study in his village because he did not want to be seen as advocating for cisgender men who have sex with men, yet he welcomed the study team conducting the study in his village inconspicuously. Another faith leader said he was aware that homosexuality existed and that if any of the study participants wished to speak to him about anything, he would welcome that exchange.

2.6.6 Institutional Review Board

In preparation for the study, the Project met with the College of Medicine Research Ethics Committee Institutional Review Board (IRB) to provide them with information related to the plight of cisgender men who have sex with men and HIV in Blantyre, Malawi. An IRB approves, monitors and reviews biomedical and behavioural research involving humans. The clinical research site staff recognized that they were inexperienced in conducting research with cisgender men who have sex with men and deemed it necessary to inform the IRB about work they had done and what they proposed for the conduct of the forthcoming study. These discussions were helpful in getting approval for the protocol of conduct to be used by the clinical research site.

2.6.7 Protocol Advisory Committee

The Protocol Advisory Committee was formed to help facilitate community engagement, gather community concerns and priorities for the study, explore the study's potential social impact, and develop responses for addressing any issues identified in collaboration with the research site's Community Advisory Board. The committee consisted of a police officer responsible for community policing, a public relations officer for Blantyre City Council, a hospital administrator, a human rights lawyer, the CAB vice-chairperson, and a staff member of CEDEP who also served on the CAB. These members were strategically selected for their support of the study and their ability to provide guidance to the site principal investigator if the study elicited negative responses. The committee also provided feedback on protocol-specific matters such as community outreach materials and the proposed study procedures. Having both a CAB and a Protocol Advisory Committee helped provide the study team with guidance necessary to implement research that required a level of caution and community mobilization above and beyond a typical feasibility study.

2.6.8 Emergency Committee

The clinical research site also established an Emergency Committee to quickly respond to potential emergency situations that might be experienced by study participants or study staff. Examples of potential emergency situations included social or physical harm to both study participants and staff, any negative media publicity, or any attempts to interfere with study implementation from the community. The Emergency Committee consisted of a study staff representative, a community liaison, and a police officer. Standard operating procedures were established by the Emergency Committee for rapid response to emergency situations. The Emergency Committee worked with CEDEP and an existing Emergency Response Centre housed in the Queen Elizabeth Central Hospital. The hospital's Emergency Response Centre provides support services to people who are victims of violence or abuse 24 h a day, 7 days a week, and includes mental health counselling, legal advice, relocation assistance, emergency medical care and police protection.

CEDEP trained the hospital's existing Emergency Response Team, as well as the clinical research site's Emergency Committee and the study staff on how to respond with cultural appropriateness when working with sexual and gender minorities who were victims of violence or abuse. The training included reflection on case scenarios to identify what constitutes an emergency and exercises on how various emergency situations can be handled. Study staff were also trained on the implementation of the emergency response standard operating procedure to ensure its implementation.

The Emergency Committee established a 24-h emergency hotline. Study staff and participants were provided the telephone number to contact in the event of any emergency, and the hotline was staffed by designated research team members. In the event of an emergency, study staff notified the Emergency Committee along with CEDEP. Study staff consulted with CEDEP as an organization that protects minority rights. Even though CEDEP had no special funding to provide support to victims of violence, they were committed to offering any housing, social or legal support possible to assist victims. The Emergency Committee worked with the hospital's Emergency Response Team to determine they type of support necessary and additional organizations that needed to be contacted to assist in an appropriate response. Any incident was also to be reported to the National Health Sciences Research and Ethics Committee within 3 days. No social harms were reported by the end of the study, but study staff reported that all the preparations were valuable because they sensitized and prepared staff for the possibility of social harm.

2.7 Recruitment

The study team used a number of strategies to recruit participants, including peer outreach and education, snowball sampling, and community sensitization training. While the study was designed to recruit cisgender men who have sex with other men, 27% of participants enrolled were born male and identified as female or transgender women. The enrolment of transgender women in the study was an unintended but important consequence of the work that opens the opportunity for additional research with subpopulations of sexual and gender minorities such as transgender women. Careful recruitment, retention, and listening enabled the study team to understand participants' varying gender identities. Crucially, the study utilized the two-step method for collection of gender identity and sex assigned at birth, without which many, if not all, of the transgender women in the study might have been miscategorized as cisgender men who have sex with men (Reisner et al., 2014).

2.7.1 Peer Outreach and Education

The Project recruited one full-time peer outreach worker whose primary responsibility was to educate and recruit cisgender men who have sex with men to the study. The outreach worker lived in one of the geographical areas from which the study team would recruit participants, so he was very familiar with the recruitment landscape. As a self-identifying gay man, he was also familiar with the study population and had established rapport with his own community.

In addition, CEDEP identified 15 peer educators who were willing to work with the outreach worker to recruit study participants. Each peer educator was assigned to one of ten geographical regions in Blantyre. Like the outreach worker, peer educators lived locally and were representative of the study population. The peer educators volunteered their time to support outreach workers on the Project as they deemed the research an important first step in securing additional research focused on cisgender men who have sex with men in Blantyre, Malawi. Some peer educators also enrolled as participants in the study, which helped to ease potential participants' concerns related to study participation and confidentiality.

> The study sounded interesting and I needed to take advantage of the medical screenings, but I was scared that some of the hospital staff would know members of my family and they would tell them that I am gay. So, I waited until other people joined to see what they would say about the study.

> My family would kick me out if they found out I was gay, and I did not want that to happen. When I found out that others were in the study and that the hospital would not tell others I was gay, I decided to join.

The outreach worker and peer educators worked with clinical research site staff to develop strategies to successfully engage participants despite the barriers of stigma and criminalization that exist in Malawi. The team developed a comprehensive outreach plan that included community sensitization and recruitment events. Peer educators identified and referred individuals who might be interested in participating in the study. They also arranged community sensitization events in their geographical region for potential study participants. At these events, the outreach worker from the Project provided information on the study.

In addition, peer educators distributed HIV prevention and treatment information and service referrals to cisgender men who have sex with men and transgender women within their assigned geographical region. These services were not part of the study but were provided through CEDEP.

2.7.2 *Snowball Sampling*

The target population in the recruitment area was known to be small and its members well connected with each other. Snowball or chain-referral sampling was therefore identified as a potentially effective recruitment strategy. Snowball sampling is a cost-effective method that can be used when recruiting members of populations who may be challenging to reach in certain environments.

Initially, this approach was not very effective because those recruited did not know what information to share with their peers to encourage them to be screened for the study. To improve participant referrals, clinic staff at the Project encouraged participants to refer others to be screened the study. Project staff provided study participants with talking points to assist with encouraging their peers to be screened. This resulted in an increase of participants referring friends and peers to be screened for the study.

2.7.3 Community Sensitization

CEDEP worked with the outreach worker and peer educators to provide community sensitization sessions at which the outreach worker could provide groups of cisgender men who have sex with men and transgender women information on HIV and AIDS, and the study. These sensitization sessions happened four times a year, and each was attended by approximately 60 individuals. They were conducted at locations outside the city of Blantyre to maintain the participants' confidentiality. Those who attended the meetings voiced some apprehension about confidentiality when participating in a study conducted by researchers unknown to the community.

> I do not know the people who are conducting this study. I know and trust the staff at CEDEP. Why aren't they conducting the study? They have conducted research in the past. Why not this study?

> How do you know these people will not tell others we are gay? This research is important, but I cannot risk others finding out I am gay.

Peer educators and the outreach worker assured session participants that safety and confidentiality were critically important to the study team. The sensitization team explained how study staff would maintain participants' confidentiality. The peer educators and outreach worker also highlighted study benefits including access to medical care and compensation for time and travel.

2.8 Retention

Retention of participants in HIV prevention research studies is vital to ensure the validity of research findings (Nyambura et al., 2014). High rates of attrition increase the risk of bias, particularly if the participants who are not retained differ from those participants who are. To achieve a high retention rate, Project staff developed a retention plan that included several strategies learned from the cultural responsiveness training provided by CEDEP. The research team held weekly staff meetings to discuss which retention strategies were working well and which needed to be revised. The most successful strategies included comprehensive locator information, a welcoming waiting area at the study site, participant retention events, and the provision of free primary health care. These strategies resulted in a retention rate overall of 86%.

2.8.1 Contact and Locator Information

Staff collected locator information for participants at the first study visit and reviewed and updated the information at each subsequent study visit. Information collected included participants' address, phone numbers, addresses and phone numbers for relatives and close friends, descriptions of locations where participants socialized, email addresses and social media contact information.

Clinic staff used the contact information to remind participants about future appointments. If a participant missed a scheduled visit, clinic staff would contact the participant and try to reschedule. If clinic staff were unsuccessful in contacting the participant, the outreach worker used the locator information collected to try to find the participant to reschedule the missed visit. The outreach worker used the clinic's nondescript study vehicle to visit locations participants provided as places they lived, worked or visited frequently.

2.8.2 *Waiting Area*

The Project provided participants with a private waiting area that included free internet, a DVD player with movies and snacks. Participants advised site staff on what DVDs to purchase for their maximum entertainment. The study staff purchased new movies every other month to bolster the video library.

2.8.3 *Transport*

Participants who enrolled in the study at the Project were provided 3000 Malawi kwacha (about US$ 4) as reimbursement for their time, effort and travel to and from the clinic for each of their study visits. For individuals who lived far from the clinic or who needed additional support for travel (i.e., because they were sick), the Project provided transportation to and from the clinic using the clinic's nondescript study vehicle.

2.8.4 *Participant Retention Events*

The study team hosted quarterly participant retention events during the study. Planned and organized by the outreach worker, activities included swimming pool parties at a local hotel and sports events. The study team rented a bus to provide transportation from the clinic to the event location. Participants could also invite friends who did not participate in the study. These events provided attendees a safe, non-judgmental space where they could live outside of the expectations of those in their community who admonished homosexuality and gender nonconformity. One participant reflected on the group's experience with these events:

> I really enjoyed the events that Johns Hopkins hosted. I liked being around my friends. It was an opportunity to be myself and not hide.

Inadvertently, these retention events also became recruitment events. While the outreach worker and peer educators would not disclose anyone's participation in the study, the participants would speak about their experiences in the study and encourage individuals who were not a part of the study to enrol.

2.8.5 Health Care

Participants who enrolled in the study received testing for HIV and STIs at each study visit. If participants had other medical concerns, they were either treated in the clinic or referred to another medical provider, depending on the issue.

Additionally, study staff also provided medical care to non-study participants who were referred to the clinic by study participants and CEDEP. These practices helped build rapport with the target populations, which resulted in participant willingness to be recruited into the study.

At the end of the study, participants were informed that funds would no longer be available for the same types of services they received during the study, but they were referred to other health care providers who would continue to provide care.

2.9 Lessons Learned

Our experience conducting this study has helped to inform the future direction of clinical trials with cisgender men who have sex with men and transgender women in sub-Saharan Africa, particularly in countries like Malawi where same-sex sexual behaviour remains a criminal offence. Studies in this context require unique approaches to stakeholder engagement, recruitment and retention. The Project learned key lessons in the following domains:

2.9.1 Stakeholder Engagement

- *Community mapping*. The Project implemented a community mapping exercise prior to the initiation of the study. This was critical to understanding the range of organizations and entities needed to engage the study population and complete enrolment and retention safely and effectively. In mapping the community, the study team found the need to engage stakeholders they had not previously considered, including law enforcement, media and community-based organizations serving sexual and gender minority populations. The exercise also helped the study team cultivate broad-based support from village chiefs, religious leaders, and government officials alike. Engaging diverse stakeholders was crucial to the success of the study and could not have been done without strategic community mapping.

- *Partnering with community-based organizations or agencies that have established rapport with study target populations.* CEDEP's expertise in serving cisgender men who have sex with men and transgender women was invaluable to the study's success. CEDEP conducted training for the study team but also helped facilitate engagement with other local stakeholders. Organizations such as CEDEP, if meaningfully involved, can assist with enrolling cisgender men who have sex with men and transgender women in similar community contexts.
- *The importance of fostering stakeholder support.* Every stakeholder the Project engaged with initially had significant concerns about the study. The study team listened to these concerns and then responded with both evidence-based and values-based messaging. The purpose of stakeholder engagement was not to change people's perspectives about homosexuality; rather, the study team persuaded stakeholders of the importance of the study as it related to community health. Over time, the clinical research site fostered buy-in from diverse stakeholders who rallied around one central message: namely, the HIV epidemic in Malawi is a public health and human rights issue that supersedes personal and political agendas. Fostering broad-based buy-in was critical to the safe and effective implementation of the study in Malawi.

2.9.2 Recruitment and Retention

- *Building trust.* By working closely with CEDEP and hosting the first community gatherings under their auspices, the study team gradually built trust among potential study participants. Staff at CEDEP, who themselves were potential study participants, were able to vouch for the study and reassure others that their safety and confidentiality were of utmost importance to the study team. Recruitment may have been less successful had the study team worked without CEDEP liaison or held community meetings in spaces perceived as less safe by the study population.
- *Utilization of snowball sampling for recruitment.* At the request of the study staff, participants encouraged their friends to enrol. The first participants already had the trust of their peers and were able to report about their positive experiences in the study. Because the study population is such a tightly knit community, participants began to enrol rapidly, as word spread from person to person within the study population.
- *The importance of listening to participants and responding to them.* The study team improved participants' experience in the study by appropriately responding to their request to upgrade their incentives. Some incentives were more meaningful to the study population than others. For example, providing transport and

basic medical health services during the study responded to the socioeconomic needs of the community and addressed the medical mistrust that is pervasive among sexual minority communities in Malawi. Hosting group outings responded to the isolation that members of the study population regularly experience.

2.10 Conclusion

Overall, the Malawi College of Medicine-Johns Hopkins University Research Project demonstrated that, with the right approach and strategic stakeholder engagement, it is possible to safely and effectively recruit sexual and gender minority populations in a country such as Malawi where same-sex behaviour is criminalized. Despite challenges in the law, barriers in religious and cultural beliefs, and difficulty gaining the trust of the study population, the Project garnered broad-based community support and successfully implement research in communities traditionally opposed to homosexuality and gender nonconformity. While the protocol was designed specifically for cisgender men who have sex with men, the Project was able to also engage and enrol transgender women. The enrolment of both cisgender men who have sex with men and transgender women in the study highlights the effectiveness of the study team's outreach and community engagement strategies, and the importance of transgender-inclusive data collection whereby gender identity and sex assigned at birth are captured. The study team used community mapping and engagement strategies to illuminate the importance of research for cisgender men who have sex with men and transgender women in ways that were meaningful and persuasive to key stakeholders. Building trust among the study population, snowball sampling and access to client-centred care enabled the clinical research site to meet its recruitment and retention goals quickly and efficiently. The success of this study in Malawi opens hopeful possibilities for much-needed future HIV prevention research with a range of sexual and gender minority populations across Africa.

References

amfAR, IAVI (International AIDS Vaccine Initiative), JHU-BSPH (Johns Hopkins Bloomberg School of Public Health), & UNDP (United Nations Development Program). (2015). *Respect, protect, fulfill: Best practices guidance in conducting HIV research with gay, bisexual, and other men who have sex with men (MSM) in rights-constrained environments*. The Foundation for AIDS Research (amfAR). Retrieved February 27, 2019, from https://www.amfar.org/uploadedFiles/_amfarorg/Articles/Around_The_World/GMT/2015/RespectProtectFulfill-MSM-ResearchGuidance-Rev2015-English.pdf

Amnesty International. (2013). *Making love a crime: Criminalization of same-sex conduct in sub-Saharan Africa*. Amnesty International Publications. Retrieved February 27, 2019, from https://www.amnestyusa.org/wp-content/uploads/2017/04/making_love_a_crime_-_africa_lgbti_report_emb_6.24.13_0.pdf

AVAC (AIDS Vaccine Advocacy Coalition), & UNAIDS (Joint United Nations Programme on HIV/AIDS). (2011). *Good participatory practice: Guidelines for biomedical HIV prevention trials*. Retrieved February 27, 2019, from https://www.avac.org/resource/good-participatory-practice-guidelines-biomedical-hiv-prevention-trials-second-edition

Ayala, G., & Santos, G.-M. (2016). Will the global HIV response fail gay and bisexual men and other men who have sex with men? *Journal of the International AIDS Society, 19*(1), 21098.

Commonwealth Lawyers Association. (2015). *The criminalization of consensual same-sex sexual relations across the commonwealth—Developments and opportunities*. Human Dignity Trust. Retrieved February 27, 2019, from https://www.humandignitytrust.org/hdt-resources/?type_filter=&tag_filter=&country_filter=&keyword_filter=criminalization+of+consensual

Fay, H., Baral, D., Trapence, G., Motimedi, F., Umar, E., Iipinge, S., Dausab, F., Wirtz, A., & Beyrer, C. (2011). Stigma, health care access, and HIV knowledge among men who have sex with men in Malawi, Namibia, and Botswana. *AIDS and Behavior, 15*(6), 1088–1097.

HIV Prevention Trials Network. (2018). Retrieved February 27, 2019, from https://hptn.org

HIV Prevention Trials Network (HPTN) 075. (2018). Retrieved February 27, 2019, from https://hptn.org/research/studies/hptn075

Nyambura, M., Otieno, F., Ndivo, R., Williamson, J., Pals, S., Mills, L., & Gust, D. A. (2014). Participant retention in a HIV prevention cohort study in Kisumu, Kenya. *Journal of Clinical Research in HIV AIDS and Prevention, 1*(4), 13–21.

Reisner, S., Biello, K., Rosenberger, J., Austin, S., Haneuse, S., Brumer, A., Perez-Brumer, A., Novak, D. S., & Mimiaga, M. J. (2014). Using a two-step method to measure transgender identity in Latin America/the Caribbean, Portugal, and Spain. *Archives of Sexual Behavior, 43* (8), 1503–1514.

Sandfort, T. G. M., Hamilton, E. L., Marais, A., Guo, X., Sugarman, J., Chen, Y. Q., Cummings, V., Dadabhai, S., Dominguez, K., Panchia, R., Schnabel, D., Zulu, F., Reynolds, D., Radebe, O., Mbeda, C., Kamba, D., Kanyemba, B., Ogendo, A., Stirratt, M., Chege, W., Lucas, J., Fawzy, M., McKinstry, L. A., & Eshleman, S. H. (2020). The feasibility of recruiting and retaining men who have sex with men and transgender women in a multinational prospective HIV prevention research cohort study in sub-Saharan Africa (HPTN 075). *Journal of the International AIDS Society, 23*, e25600.

UNAIDS (Joint United Nations Programme on HIV/AIDS). (2016). *Prevention gap report*. UNAIDS. Retrieved January 5, 2021, from http://www.unaids.org/sites/default/files/media_asset/2016-prevention-gap-report_en.pdf

UNAIDS (Joint United Nations Programme on HIV/AIDS). (2017). *UNAIDS data book 2017*. UNAIDS. Retrieved February 27, 2019, from http://www.unaids.org/sites/default/files/media_asset/20170720_Data_book_2017_en.pdf

Wirtz, A., Trapence, G., Kamba, D., Gama, V., Chalera, R., Jumbe, V., Kumwenda, R., Mangochi, M., Helleringer, S., Beyrer, C., & Baral, S. (2017). Geographical disparities in HIV prevalence and care among men who have sex with men in Malawi: Results from a multisite cross-sectional survey. *The Lancet HIV, 4*(6), 206–269.

Chapter 3
"Heavy Drinking" and HIV Vulnerability Among African Male Sex Workers: Narratives from a Community-Based Participatory Study in Nairobi, Kenya

Robert Lorway, Monika Doshi, John Mathenge, Pascal Macharia, Lyle McKinnon, Parinita Bhattacharjee, Helgar K. Musyoki, Akram Pasha, Lisa Lazarus, Sushena Reza-Paul, Joshua Kimani, and Matthew Thomann

With growing attention to the vulnerability of men who have sex with men in African contexts to HIV, public health scientists and others have begun to draw

R. Lorway (✉) · P. Bhattacharjee · L. Lazarus
Institute for Global Public Health, Department of Community Health Sciences, University of Manitoba, Winnipeg, MB, Canada
e-mail: Robert.Lorway@umanitoba.ca

M. Doshi
School of Public Health, University of Michigan, Ann Arbor, MI, USA

J. Mathenge · P. Macharia
Health Options for Young Men on HIV/AIDS & STIs (HOYMAS), Nairobi, Kenya

L. McKinnon
Department of Medical Microbiology, University of Manitoba, Winnipeg, MB, Canada
e-mail: Lyle.Mckinnon@umanitoba.ca

H. K. Musyoki
Kenya National AIDS & STI Control Programme (NASCOP), Ministry of Health, Nairobi, Kenya
e-mail: helgar@nascop.or.ke

A. Pasha
Ashodaya Samithi, Mysore, Karnataka, India

S. Reza-Paul
Institute for Global Public Health, Department of Community Health Sciences, University of Manitoba, Winnipeg, MB, Canada

Ashodaya Samithi, Mysore, Karnataka, India

J. Kimani
Department of Medical Microbiology, University of Nairobi, Nairobi, Kenya
e-mail: Jkimani@csrtkenya.org

M. Thomann
Department of Anthropology, University of Maryland, College Park, MD, USA

T. Sandfort (ed.), *Male Same-sex Sexuality and HIV in Sub-Saharan Africa*, Social Aspects of HIV 7, https://doi.org/10.1007/978-3-030-73726-9_3

connections between alcohol use in this population and the transmission of HIV and other sexually transmitted infections. In this chapter, we consider the role of the global health discourse in shaping the meanings, experiences, and subjectivities of male sex workers in Kenya with respect to heavy drinking, referred to locally in Kiswahili as kulewa (getting drunk). Employing a community-based participatory research approach, we conducted in-depth interviews with male sex workers ($n = 41$) in Nairobi, Kenya. Our findings illuminate how drinking narratives are influenced by regionally based HIV interventions. Global health discourse, we contend, (1) constructs the sexual health of male sex workers as continually 'in jeopardy' while it (2) compels male sex workers to reflect on and enact ways to improve 'community health.' We describe how male sex workers rework reigning global health discourses that reduce problem drinking to 'poor' individual decision making. Instead, their narratives depict heavy drinking as tied to multiple overlapping oppressions faced by a wider community of male sex workers.

> One of the biggest mistakes that we [male sex workers] do is alcohol . . . . We end up messing [up] a lot; because when you are *uko maji* [intoxicated], some precautions that you are supposed to take, you never take them. And that's why we end up getting so many diseases. Alcohol… leads us even to stealing…leads us to fights. For me, if I want a good date, I drink. You go, the two of you, have a few drinks and go do what you are supposed to do [have sex], and part your own ways. But when it comes to a crowd where you are drinking you end up *kunywa pombe nyingi* [drinking too much alcohol] . . . I mean you will not even remember to use a condom. That is one thing I know alcohol is. It affects the sex workers—yeah, it does affect you and you end up losing a lot. You lose your money in the process. You end up being abused because you were drunk; somebody beats you up and leaves you there.

In this chapter, we examine the socio-cultural linkages between heavy drinking—referred to as "hazardous drinking" in the public health literature (see for example: Knox et al., 2017)—and the sexual health of a group of African men who have sex with men. More specifically, as a case study, we analyse a set of narratives generated through a participatory action research project conducted by male sex workers leading a vibrant community-based organization in Nairobi and undertaken in collaboration with a team of Kenyan and Canadian health researchers. These narratives illuminate the various associations that male sex workers themselves draw in relation to heavy drinking—associations that locate what is known in local Kiswahili as *kulewa* (getting drunk) at the heart of various social and structural problems their community contends with in their daily lives. Although these narratives frequently frame heavy drinking as leading to forms of abuse, as the quotation above suggests, in our analysis we avoid a simplistic interpretation of these narratives that would reduce them to individualistic "perceptions" or traumatized psychological states. Our attempt is not to diminish the experiential realities related to heavy drinking, which certainly trouble male sex workers. Instead, by drawing upon anthropological perspectives, we aim to provide a broader analytic framework for understanding heavy drinking among male sex workers than public health depictions currently furnish.

With growing attention on the health and human rights of gay, bisexual, and other men who have sex with men in African contexts over the last decade (see for example: Baral et al., 2009), public health scientists and others have begun to explore connections between their use of alcohol and the transmission of HIV and other sexual transmitted infections (STIs) (Kalichman et al., 2007; Knox et al., 2017; Lane et al., 2008, 2011; Parry et al., 2008; Van der Elst et al., 2013). Health scientists have conducted various quantitative behavioural studies in urban centres of Kenya among this group to assess the prevalence and frequency of alcohol consumption (McKinnon et al., 2014; Muraguri et al., 2015), while employing clinical psychological scales to capture levels of alcohol dependency and draw statistical associations with unprotected anal sex (Geibel et al., 2008, 2012). These epidemiologically oriented findings echo public health concerns over alcohol use and the HIV vulnerability of men who have sex with men throughout Africa (Sandfort et al., 2017) and worldwide (Purcell et al., 2001). Although a handful of important qualitative studies do mention alcohol use in relation to the sexual practices of men who have sex with men in Kenya (for example see Okal et al., 2009), we know far less about the sociocultural circumstances in which drinking practices occur within these communities and how alcohol consumption takes shape within wider political economic fields of power (Singer, 1986).

Earlier cross-cultural anthropological studies of "drunkenness" challenge commonly held negative assumptions around drinking by treating it as a cultural construct that is "woven into the very fabric of social existence" (Marshall, 1979, p. 2). However, this approach eventually came under fire as rendering a functionalist narrative that overemphasized the beneficial aspects of drinking as socially integrative (Room, 1984). In his foundational essay, medical anthropologist Merrill Singer (1986) rightly criticizes overly relativistic ethnographic accounts of drinking by advocating, instead, for a world-systems approach that places drinking and social life in a political economic view. The historian Justin Willis (2002) offers such a perspective in his study of East African social patterns of "temperance" and "drunkenness", in which he examines the shifting moral value of alcohol in relation to traditional authority, colonialism, and postcolonial preoccupations with modernity. Although offering a vital backdrop for interpreting current alcohol consumption in the region, Willis's historical rendition holds limited insight for helping make sense of male sex workers' interpretations of heavy drinking. Their experiences of alcohol consumption are increasingly shaped by western-funded HIV interventions and other incursions into their sexual health and human rights. Because such intervention by countries in the global North are met with postcolonial, nationalist discourses, male sex workers' experiences of alcohol are entangled in much broader discourses of authenticity and belonging.

Building on this political economic perspective, we consider the vital role of a global health apparatus in shaping meanings, experiences, and subjectivities with respect to drinking. This global health apparatus capitalizes on previous "LGBT rights" mobilizations across the African continent that stirred identity politics in the 1990s around anti-homosexual government rhetoric. African LGBT rights organizing already "responsibilized" (Ilcan & Basok, 2004) groupings of sexual dissidents to become the custodians of social justice projects. Today, these rights-based collectives persist alongside global health programmes, and many have coalesced into "hybrid organizations, addressing a combination of public-health and social-justice issues raised by their diverse constituents" (Currier & McKay, 2017, p. 75).

The global health apparatus, we contend, is influential in how it simultaneously (1) constructs the sexual health of male sex workers as continually 'in jeopardy' while it (2) compels male sex workers to reflect on and enact ways to improve and safeguard 'community health.' We contextualize their heavy drinking narratives by emphasizing the collective engagements of a group of male sex workers who actively confront what they have come to identify as threats to their collective health and wellbeing.

Currently, health scientists working on HIV programmes for men who have sex with men who contend with drinking problems tend to recommend individual-centred "risk reduction counselling" or cognitive behavioural therapy (for example see Taegtmeyer et al., 2013; Coates et al., 2013). The complexity invoked in participants' narratives of *kulewa*, we argue, not only offers vivid insight into how heavy drinking undermines the effectiveness of existing HIV prevention and treatment programmes, but also gestures toward the environmental and structural conditions that need to be considered to mitigate heavy drinking and more holistically improve the wellbeing of this community.

3.1 The Emergence of a Global Health Apparatus

Historically, epidemiologists have classified parts of Africa as having a "generalized" or "pattern II (heterosexual)" epidemic because of high HIV prevalence appearing among people who were viewed as not fitting within the early HIV risk group models employed in the West (Treichler, 1999). The "invention of African AIDS", to borrow Cindy Patton's (1990) words, gave rise to the idea of a "heterosexual epidemic" that could be regarded as distinctive from Euro-American epidemics primarily affecting gay men. This notion fed into and reinforced stereotypical ideas of African sexuality as monolithically heterosexual (Patton, 1990). UNAIDS and WHO statistics in the 1980s, 1990s and early 2000s indeed reflected the assumed lack of sexual diversity in African populations in their portrayal of HIV sexual transmission between African men as contributing "0%" to new infections. This portrayal of heterosexual uniformity and non-transmission appeared all the more curious amid highly visible emerging LGBT social movements that organized across various African nations in response to vilifying government rhetoric that cast homosexuality as an imported European cultural practice that threatened the integrity of African nation states (Awondo, 2010; Currier, 2012; Lorway et al., 2014; Ndjio, 2012; Nyanzi, 2013). Many African LGBT leaders during this period called for greater attention to be paid to their HIV prevention and care needs but were largely ignored by public health (Johnson & Cameron, 2007).

Shattering the epidemiologic construction of Africa's "heterosexual epidemic", Baral et al. (2009) demonstrated that HIV, in fact, was transmitted between men who had sex with men in southern Africa, as evidenced by alarmingly high HIV prevalence in this group. Subsequent epidemiologic studies further unsettled the distinction assumed to exist between generalized and concentrated epidemics with the identification of high HIV prevalence among "key populations" (e.g., sex workers, people who inject drugs, and men who have sex with men) in supposed "generalized epidemics settings" in Africa (Baral et al., 2014; Tanser et al., 2014).

The realization of elevated susceptibility among men who have sex with men in Africa marked a dramatic shift in global funding priorities for HIV prevention, treatment, and care. When the US President's Plan for Emergency Relief (PEPFAR) began in 2004, very little information on the HIV vulnerability of men who have sex with men in Africa existed. However, as high HIV prevalence among men who have sex with men came to light between 2006 and 2008, PEFAR began to fund and push for increased bio-behavioural surveillance within these populations, in Southern and Eastern Africa (Needle et al., 2012). At the time of writing, PEPFAR serves as the major funding source for HIV prevention, treatment, and care among men who have sex with men in many African countries. This policy shift brings together diverse, transnational consortia of health actors including multilateral representatives, government health officials, academics and health scientists, and local health professionals—by the epidemiological expertise and policies of the US Centers for Disease Control and Prevention (CDC)—to design programmes that deliver specialized health services to men who have sex with men in African countries. Within this epistemic community, the mantra of "community mobilization" intensified around efforts to reach those considered to be hidden so as to increase their uptake of health services. Anthropologist Elsa Fan (2014, p. 86) notes the global trend in which community-based organizations led by men who have sex with men become drawn into the outsourcing of health service provision. Similarly, specialized clinical services throughout Kenya emphasized ideologies of "community mobilization" and encouraged the formation of local collectives to ensure the steady flow of STI patients to meet targets prescribed by PEFAR-CDC funders (see also Lorway, 2017).

3.2 The Formation of HOYMAS

On September 18, 2009, 14 male sex workers living in Nairobi officially registered their collective, known as Health Options for Young Men on HIV/AIDS and STIs (HOYMAS), as a community-based organization with the Kenyan Ministry of Gender & Social Services (Lorway, 2017). The collective began as a social support group that sought to protect their members from violence, provide care for those who were ill, and lend money to those struggling to subsist. Initially, the founding members of the community-based organization met in public places such as bars, parks and other locations where they conducted sex work (see Igonya & Moyer, 2016 for a compelling and more detailed ethnographic account of the emergence of care and support in this community).

When the first author initially met the founders of HOYMAS in early 2009, staff had begun to hold regular meetings in the boardroom of a specialized sex worker clinic in Nairobi known as SWOP (Sex Workers Outreach Project)—a programme managed jointly by the universities of Nairobi and Manitoba. SWOP's health services were originally set up to attract female sex workers; yet when men selling sex presented at the clinic with high rates of HIV infection and other STIs, the clinical team began to expand the services they offered to include men. SWOP soon secured PEPFAR funding to track and follow the health status of male sex workers. At the outset, HOYMAS quickly filled a major gap in health services by providing vital support and health education to sex work clients and sex worker peers (Lorway, 2017). HOYMAS also aided the efforts of SWOP clinicians to assemble a male sex worker cohort, a study which eventually found extremely high HIV and STI prevalence and incidence (McKinnon et al., 2014). This cohort of more than 500 people further enlarged the organization's membership base and soon national AIDS policy entities such as NASCOP (the National AIDS and STIs Control Programme) began to endorse the community-based organization as a model programme for East Africa. In many ways, then, the organization emerged as a "biosocial collective" (Rabinow & Rose, 2006), continually transforming in relation to their collaborative HIV work with allied clinical scientists, counsellors and national health officials.

Despite this HIV-specific support, as Igonya (2017) notes, male sex workers in Nairobi also frequently criticize transnationally mediated HIV interventions in the region for failing to recognize the more pressing concerns of the community around their low incomes and ongoing human rights violations. Although anchored to sexual health campaigns tied to particular global health logics of outsourcing and "bioexperimentalism" (Lorway, 2017, p. 108), the HOYMAS collective continually pushed against the biomedical strictures that conceived of their well-being in primarily epidemiological terms by initiating a number of social justice initiatives. For instance, in February 2014 HOYMAS welcomed asylum seekers fleeing impending discrimination in Uganda when a tabloid newspaper there published the names of "200 top homosexuals", following President Museveni's approval of anti-homosexual legislation further penalizing Ugandans. In December 2017, HOYMAS held a peaceful march in the Central Business District of Nairobi to recognize International Day to End Violence Against Sex Workers, gathering together more than 500 male and female sex workers to raise public awareness and address the news media. Therefore, in addition to daily health service delivery commitments and regular interactions with health professionals and scientists, HOYMAS staff and many of its members actively participated in LGBT and sex worker alliances and political forums, thereby continually blurring the dividing lines between health and human rights interests in ways that grounded global health ideologies in the daily lived concerns of their membership.

3.3 South-to-South Collaborations

During the 2012 boycotting of the International AIDS Conference in Washington, DC, which excluded sex workers (and substance users) who were unable to obtain visas, the director of HOYMAS, the third author, connected with the leaders of a sex work collective based in South India, known as *Ashodaya Samithi* (Lorway, 2017). Following the fortuitous meeting in Kolkata, he travelled to Mysore to view Ashodaya's programmes. There he, in conversation with the first author, expressed how deeply impressed he was by how the community was running the programmes and how Ashodaya exerted influence over clinical services (Dixon et al., 2012). As a prominent sex worker activist in Nairobi, the third author also became interested in the community research projects that Ashodaya had led over the years in Mysore (see for example: Lorway et al., 2009).

After his return to Kenya, the director approached the first author with the idea of conducting a participatory action research project in collaboration with Ashodaya so that "the research questions, data collection, interpretations and recommendations would be driven by the experiences, interests and insights of the male sex work community in Nairobi" (Lorway, 2017). Around the same time, a Kenyan scientist who led the male sex worker cohort study at SWOP approached the first author to discuss the HIV-related health problems afflicting the male sex workers enrolled in his study. At baseline, the 510 cohort participants showed a 40% HIV prevalence; within a year, 12% of the uninfected men tested positive for HIV (McKinnon et al., 2014). The scientist expressed his exasperation, for their team had provided condoms and lubricants, HIV risk reduction counselling, and HIV prevention education—yet the seroconversion rate remained extremely high.

Eventually HOYMAS and the Kenyan scientist united their concerns and became co-investigators on the eventual research project, funded by the Canadian Institutes of Health Research, while they nominated the first author, a medical anthropologist, as the principal investigator. This research collaboration brought together sex workers and health scientists from Kenya, India, and Canada to form a project that operated on the assumption that the priorities, perspectives, and experiential knowledge of male sex workers needed to be more forcefully positioned within existing Kenyan policymaking arenas concerned with their health and well-being.

3.4 Participant Recruitment and Training

HOYMAS staff selected ten community leaders from the male sex work community to serve as interviewers and researcher supervisors. This community research team, comprised of male sex workers, were selected from various demographic and sexual network backgrounds (i.e., according to age, socio economic status, and location of sex work) to allow them to recruit a diverse study sample. There were three training sessions: first to discuss research ethics, interview guide development, and to learn interviewing techniques; second, to learn about and practice interpretive and content analysis techniques; and third to build skills around preparing and delivering oral presentations for the eventual dissemination of the study findings to county and national policy makers.

Community research team members were trained to ask qualitative interview questions effectively, mirroring a methodology described elsewhere (Lorway et al., 2014). The community researchers were also asked to identify themes related to their community's intense HIV vulnerability. The themes they identified included both health and human rights. The interview guide included the following questions about human rights: (1) "Are you aware of your rights as a male sex worker? If "Yes", can you tell me what you know about your rights?"; (2) "In case your rights are violated, how would you deal with that?", and (3) "What are your thoughts and feelings about male sex workers publicly demonstrating for their rights?" This chapter focuses on a subset of questions focused on alcohol consumption ("What do you know about alcohol use among male sex workers?" and "Can you talk about any experiences you have had using alcohol, including problems that using alcohol has created for you?"), which elicited richly detailed narratives from the community researchers' peers.

3.5 Research Training Challenges

The research training process, which engaged community leaders at discrete intervals over a 2-year period, offered a vivid window into some of the struggles that male sex workers regularly face. Although the training was generally well attended, various problems impeded the sessions at times. Two trainees, on different occasions, were unable to attend a training session because they had been arrested and imprisoned as part of regular police sweeps in the downtown centre where they were soliciting clients in the evening. We halted the training those days so that HOYMAS staff could advocate for their release, which was successful. Two other community researchers had problems keeping a place of residence because of their inability to pay rent on time, and therefore they had difficulty making a few of the training sessions. Another leader at times struggled to participate because he had persistent health problems. He avoided seeking medical attention because he was concerned about the cost of health services. A HOYMAS staff member discussed the issues with the first and second author (who were leading the training) and explained that many of these problems were related to pervasive alcohol dependency in the community. As research trainers, we also learned about the pervasiveness of problem drinking in relation to the travel per diems regularly provided to training participants. Although these modest funds accumulated over time, many of the trainees continued to be left without any money for rent, food and the ability to pay for health services (that fell outside of the PEPFAR- CDC-funded free clinical system); and some arrived at the training sessions each day progressively more intoxicated. The HOYMAS director eventually recommended the adjustment of the administration of training per diems. In collaboration with the community researchers, HOYMAS decided that a portion of the per diem should be paid for a yearly health insurance plan and, for the community researchers who struggled to keep a stable residence, they agreed that the community-based organization would safeguard a portion of their payment until rent was due.

3.6 Participant Demographics

A total of 41 male sex workers were interviewed. Close to half of the participants were not enrolled in the health programmes offered by HOYMAS, although they were still closely tied to the community-based organization through its extensive health outreach networks. Three-quarters of the participants were between 18 and 34 years of age. Nearly half of the participants reported being single or never married and over one-quarter reported being married. Among those married, over one-half reported being married to a man; a union that is not legally recognized in Kenya. All participants reported having exposure to formal education, with the majority having finished secondary school. Moreover, a significant proportion of the participants were well-educated as nearly two-thirds reported having completed either technical/ vocational training or university. Despite work-force readiness, the Kenyan economy has been unable to engage new entrants into productive employment. Youth unemployment is estimated to be as high as 35% and approximately 80% of unemployed Kenyans are between 15 and 34 years of age (Zepeda et al., 2013). The extent to which ongoing discrimination endured by Kenyan male sex workers further inhibits their chances of entering other forms of employment (beyond sex work) requires further research.

Over three-quarters of the participants reported that their main source of income was from sex work. Among those who reported sex work as the primary source of income, nearly two-thirds reported a secondary source of income to supplement earnings from sex work. Of those participants who reported a primary income source other than sex work, nearly four-fifths reported relying on sex work as supplementary/secondary source of income. Supplementary income sources, when not sex work, usually included petty businesses or employment in community-led health initiatives, such as HOYMAS, which often rely on international donor funding to support their administrative and labour infrastructure costs.

3.7 Heavy Drinking

Participants often narrated the problems they associated with heavy drinking by invoking "the community" rather than speaking of their individual experience. This discursive practice speaks to the solidarity they shared with each other—that is, a sense of social belonging cultivated by HOYMAS via their health and social justice projects. Long before the interviews, community researchers told the first author that issues around alcohol had already been discussed, at great length, during health promotion workshops organized by their community-based organization. Having observed some of these workshops prior to data collection, the first author witnessed how HOYMAS members negotiated and generated collective meanings that drew linkages between alcohol use, HIV vulnerability, social and economic problems, and human rights denials with respect to homosexuality and sex work. These forms of collective narration were reflected in the tone and content of the interview narratives produced during the qualitative study. Many of the narratives take on an "advice-giving" quality, which was often directed at the wider male sex work community, thereby aligning with the education messaging that imbued HOYMAS' community health promotion work. The way that narratives repeatedly employed acronyms, such as "MSM" (men who have sex with men) and "MSW" (male sex workers) and made reference to "PEP" (post-exposure prophylaxis) and anti-retroviral medication in relation to heavy alcohol use also signified how particular public health ideas had become socially embedded in their community. This also held true among participants not enrolled in HOYMAS's health programmes. Because they were tied to HOYMAS through its outreach networks, their narratives too were highly influenced by health intervention discourses targeting "the community".

3.7.1 Reasons for Drinking

Participants consistently portrayed alcohol use as a normal and even obligatory part of doing their work, particularly because sex work took place in venues that sold alcohol.

> Okay in this industry there is always use of alcohol. . . . [S]o it is a normal thing, because me I get my clients from a club and you don't expect somebody like me going to a club and taking a soda or something. So, like you have to take alcohol. (George,[1] 22 years)

In bars and nightclubs where male sex workers commonly solicited clients and connected with their peers, alcohol mediated their social interactions. Many participants felt that their clients expected them to consume alcohol, as their work involved "partying" with clients.

Most participants asserted that heavy drinking was one of the most serious problems facing their community, and portrayed alcohol as an integral part of the community's suffering. At the same time, they frequently attached contradictory meanings to alcohol use with respect to sex work. Many participants claimed that the psychoactive effects of alcohol offered some benefit by enabling them to cope with the stress arising from their unequal social positioning.

> The key point here is, you see, people who sell sex. . . . you will find the MSW in bars drinking. Do you know why? There is somebody who was evicted from their home, he is stressed. Another one just found out they are [HIV] positive, he drinks to reduce the stress. You also get your clients in the bar, because that is the hotspot. Yeah, so you have to take alcohol for you to manipulate yourself to feel . . . to avoid stigma. (Sam, 28 years)

During group analysis, the community researchers explained that alcohol enabled their peers to manage the multiple layers of shame they endured as a community. "Internalized stigma", as some community researchers called it, was attached to the

[1]All the names used are pseudonyms.

act of having sex with another man and intensified by selling sex. The layers of shame that male sex workers encountered, according to the community researchers, arose in their families, in their community or "tribe", and at a national level with regard to the anti-gay statements made during parliamentary debates in Kenya. Alcohol was viewed as a form of self-medication against the distress associated with daily social stigma.

As the following quotation illustrates, drinking also helped participants to cope with the emotional toll they felt in having sex with multiple partners on a given day.

> First of all, someone takes alcohol to remove the guilt. You know at times you just sit thinking about something you did, that didn't please you while... selling sex. So, you just take alcohol to remove the thoughts, to let the pain go off a bit. Then another reason is to handle clients; you know, per day you can't, there's no way you can handle two, three, four or more than that when you are sober.... You don't see it as wrong because *uko maji* [you are intoxicated]. (David, 30 years)

Another participant attributed their suffering to the criminalized status of sex work, a problem which they felt alcohol helped to ease.

> Oh, if there is something they do every day [it] is alcohol; because one thing, you know this thing [sex work] is not legal in the first place. And again, doing it with people who are ... psychologically affected or maybe they have problems with their marriages, maybe they're bisexuals, you know, you can find yourself in problems. So what we do is that we spend a lot in drinking. (Jeff, 23 years)

Participant narratives often depicted alcohol as providing disinhibition to overcome social stigma to have sex with their clients. In other words, they relied upon the psychophysiological effects of alcohol to do their work. The notion of only being able to have sex with another man while under the influence of alcohol was a *Leitmotif* that ran across the narratives.

> It is very common. And I was once in that group [of male sex workers] and I would not sex up with a man without alcohol, that was my motto; no alcohol, no sex, whether client or not. (Erick, 33 years)

> You know... [if] he [a hypothetical client] doesn't drink alcohol; he can't make love to another man. If he doesn't drink alcohol; if you don't give him alcohol you won't know his secret.... Now it's how he was created. You see? He will tell you yes, I'm gay, but if you don't give me alcohol, I can't go with you. [Only after he consumed alcohol] if you go with him in bed, he will strip all your clothes. (Michael, 39 years)

What emerges from these narratives is the notion that alcohol, and its psychoactive effects of disinhibition, in the context of deeply embedded stigma, is crucial for both male sex workers and clients to cope with stigma and to express their erotic desires. Because homosexuality was viewed as culturally forbidden, alcohol was a necessary preface to having sex. During group exercises that contextualized the findings, the community researchers further explained that the way their community practiced sex work was quite different from their female colleagues. They insisted that the sexual interactions of male sex workers with clients tended to be less business-like than those of female sex workers, often blurring the lines between a mercantile and an intimate social relationship. Importantly, this explanation is consistent with what is known about male sex work cross-culturally (Aggleton & Parker, 2014). Within the context of male sex work, men not only earn or supplement their income by selling sex, but they also explore their sexual desires in ways that often dissolve the clear dividing line assumed to exist between "a client" and "a sexual partner."

Many participants regarded approaching prospective clients or other sexual partners, within the context of intense social stigmatization, as a daunting task that was anxiety inducing. Much of this anxiety centred around the uncertainty of the sexual preference of a potential client or partner, and the negative consequences when making an incorrect assumption around a potential client's sexual interest. However, the relaxing physiological effect of alcohol was understood by participants as giving them the necessary courage to approach potential clients.

> [Alcohol] eliminates fear.... Because there is someone you want; but telling them, you will not be able to. And you know he is [sexually attracted to men] and you know you are, but how to tell him is hard. But when I take one bottle and the second, even *chang'aa* [a very cheap and strong traditional brew of alcohol], if it's one glass, I drink the second. Now when you start like this, I will come and tell you. And I don't care how you will take it. One [potential client] will insult you, another will just keep quiet, and yes it has that advantage. (Joseph, 44 years)

> Yes, sometimes you feel like quitting alcohol but there's a time when it comes when you need it no matter what. I need to go out to work, I need to look for men, I need to eat and I have to be out tonight. So, I have to get something to loosen me up...most of the times I go *nikiwa madre* [when I'm high]. Because I can feel uh...I can, I can talk to like anybody, I won't feel scared by city *askaris* [municipal police force], uh...my mind will be just easy...Yeah, I won't fear, I won't fear. (Peter, 30 years)

3.7.2 Loss and Losing Control

The effects of heavy drinking, according to the majority of the participants, were associated with the notion of "loss": the loss of material items, like cell phones, cash and other possessions; loss of employment, clients, and earnings; and loss of one's sense of agency. Participant narratives of drunkenness especially depicted the male sex workers as losing control over their own financial situation—unable to save from their sex work earnings and causing some to stop drinking all together.

> So basically, MSMs get money but they misuse the money via alcohol. Instead of raising their living standards, they spend it all on alcohol abuse yeah....okay basically alcohol is bad because of first you waste your finances; you know, we are sex workers and basically as MSMs or rather as male sex workers we don't have, we don't meet clients daily but after some time unlike the female sex workers who can meet like ten clients daily. So, think of a situation when a MSM meets a client, he parts with 10,000 KES [$97USD] and drops himself in a pub....comes the following morning he has no coin in his pocket. So, I just felt like I was wasting much [of the] funds that I had, and decided to stop [drinking] because it was not benefitting; instead I was losing a lot yeah. (Erick, 33 years)

Participants recounted sexual encounters of heavy drinking that led to black-outs or periods of memory loss.

> You just go with anyone, cause you are drunk, you don't know what you are doing, you don't know who you are going with, you are just letting go. What happened is that I went to, I didn't even know the place. Yeah, when I woke up, it's the moment I am only realizing 'My God this is not the place that I am used to' yeah... not even somebody that I don't even know; somebody that I didn't give myself out to. (Bernard, 22 years)

Of particular concern to participants was how such memory loss could lead to unprotected sex.

> Because this bad situation, I found myself in was that I had unprotected sex [with a client]. I was drunk and we went to sleep, I found out that we had engaged in sex without using the condom. So that is a bad situation that I found myself in. I, on reaching the next morning, I saw that I had engaged in sex without using the condom. That is when I rushed to the hospital for help [to obtain PEP] again. So that is a situation that I was in. Yes. (Stephen, 32 years)

> We had gone to have fun at a particular event; it was a match, a rugby match at Machakos [a sports arena]. So ... we went with my friends and had fun, had fun. . .getting drunk, doing things you don't do at your normal state. So basically, after we got drunk, I got drunk and blacked out, so after blacking out I can't tell you what happened. But all and all I know I had sex with a guy [a client] ... after some weeks I started having some STI symptoms ... I went to the hospital... it hit me, damn, I have an STI because I was, my mind was intoxicated. I mean I drank alcohol. (David, 30 years)

Heavy drinking was also held responsible for scenarios in which clients took financial advantage of male sex workers and often in tandem with scenarios of involuntary unprotected sex.

> I found myself sleeping with someone and he didn't give me money he just left ten shillings [$0.10USD]. ... And the house I slept in was for twelve hundred shillings [$11.65USD] per night. ... We went to a club, we drank and drank, I don't know what I did I got completely drunk and slept. I found myself in bed, am naked, condoms are on the floor, and it's not even two or three. Waking up I found ten shillings on the table. When I called him he insulted me and hanged up. So, from there I knew alcohol is not good. (Simon, 21 years)

> I can say that alcohol has ruined my life totally. ... If I get a client, he starts buying you alcohol, you get totally drunk. When you go to a room you are not even able to negotiate well about the payments so you find that the client maybe has under-paid you; maybe you were supposed to ask for 2,000 KES [$19.42USD], he has just left 200 KES [$1.94USD] for you and you are not even aware that if you used condom. In the morning you can't even tell if he used condom or not and again you also forget that you are supposed to take your drugs [antiretrovirals]. So alcohol has really done a lot of harm. (Chris, 26 years)

The theme of loss of control also featured prominently in participants' discussions of drunkenness and sexual assault. Although only a couple of participants claimed to have actually been gang raped, the idea of such sexual violence troubled many of the narratives of heavy drinking.

> One [friend who is a male sex worker] was drinking alcohol and he had a *bleki* [slang for black out] and he got gang raped. The next thing before he knew it, he found himself in Nairobi in hospital, some good Samaritans took him there because after these guys, they gang raped him, they threw him in a trench because they obviously didn't care, they didn't even have that humane of at least taking him to hospital no they did not do that. Then, too, he found himself infected with HIV already. ... Infected and it was terrible for him actually he took a lot of time to heal you know? To heal in the mind; it was too traumatic. (Ian, 32 years)

Instead of responding to the questions around problem drinking by providing a personal narrative, many of the participants instead chose to respond by generalizing heavy drinking as a community health problem, while others offered advice to their peers.

> To my fellow male sex workers I would tell them it is not advisable to take alcohol when you are selling sex because when you take alcohol and you are having sex or maybe you are having so many clients not just one client at a night, maybe you are having two, three clients it is not advisable because you can forget maybe to put on a condom and maybe you don't know this client health wise so you can get infected by STIs and maybe even HIV/AIDS. (Martin, 24 years)

> Well I try my best to tell them [other male sex workers] not to drink a lot because if you go and have sex with somebody and you are drunk, this person may take advantage of you, he may not use condom, he may have sex with you and leave without paying you. (Brian, 22 years)

Important to note here is how many of the narratives take on the moral tone of a warning to the broader male sex worker community. This expression of concern for "the community" can be linked to the environment created by HOYMAS. Having observed some of HOYMAS' health promotion sessions, it became clear to the first author that their programmes sought to cultivate a communal sense of responsibility, tied to the collective social justice pursuits of the organization.

3.8 Heavy Drinking and HIV Vulnerability

3.8.1 Alcohol, Post-exposure Prophylaxis and Antiretrovirals

The problems that participants attributed to heavy drinking suggested a downward spiral toward HIV vulnerability. Loss of control, blacking out, violation of consent, unprotected sex, and social and financial ruin suggested the inescapable jeopardy of the community. When heavy drinking narratives recounted unprotected sexual encounters, the stories often came to an abrupt dénouement when participants made a visit to the clinic for post-exposure prophylaxis (PEP)—a kind of "morning after" pill (i.e., an antiretroviral, or ARV) prescribed to prevent HIV infection.

> There is a time I was introduced to a friend and we went and drank and after that we went and booked a room. We had agreed we were going to have sex. . .we had discussed protection as well. The guy was totally drunk and when we had sex, I realized that he had taken off the condom, he had fucked me without a condom, and we had agreed on using the condom. So personally, I think there is a big problem with having sex while drunk.

> I felt very bad, but I couldn't do anything because he had already taken it off. He took it off immediately and got into me without it. I came to realize it after we had finished.. . .I thought of reporting it to the police, but that didn't work. I felt that if I went to the police, that would make matters worse for me, I could even be deemed at fault and jailed. Because I know men having sex with other men is illegal. After that, I felt that the best thing was to let it go. I went to hospital and was given some medication [PEP] but I hadn't contracted any disease. Yeah. (Martin, 24 years)

> The problem I had was one time I was with a client, but that time I was still negative, so I went for PEP and I was given. Now the next time, the same thing happened because I was drunk. When I went to the clinic they told to make sure I use condoms and lube so that I stop going for PEP all the time. That time I did not have lube, I used to use saliva and then the condom burst because of the friction. The third time when I went for PEP, they told me that they would test me first and that was when they found I had HIV. (Patrick, 23 years)

Participants expressed considerable distress around the perceived relationship between heavy drinking and unprotected sex—an understandable concern for people living in a context of extremely high HIV prevalence. Participants enrolled in HOYMAS programmes were acutely aware of this reality through the various HIV educational workshops they attended. Although these participants had ready access to PEP as a safety precaution after such encounters, their stories made little mention of how the risk reduction counselling they received along with PEP enabled them to avoid this vulnerability in the future.

Furthermore, participants living with HIV repeatedly drew associations between heavy drinking and missing their scheduled ARV dosage.

> Well, I can give you one issue. It's not the first time, it has happened about three times now, that after I drink alcohol, I don't remember to take my medicines. That is why I am saying that alcohol is not good for people living with HIV because once you get drunk you don't remember to take your medicine, you normally remember the next day, that oh, yesterday I didn't take my medicine. Also to people living with HIV, a lot of alcohol is not good. Even if you drink, don't drink too much. Drink on maybe just one day in a week, that you can be okay, instead of taking it every day, where you won't even get the time to take your medicines. (Moses, 32 years)

> We drink to an extent of passing out. Let's say you are positive, and you stayed in the club and you got drunk and you slept; the time for your [ARV] medication, you won't even take.... There was a time especially like me when I was drinking alcohol, even if I was taking medicine I couldn't take. Even if it's food I couldn't eat... Now I continue taking alcohol. But telling me to sit and eat, even that appetite I didn't have it. So drinking alcohol is not good to people like us. First of all, you will *not swallow your medicine*, secondly you won't eat food, and thirdly you won't use protection because it's just alcohol that is in your head and it shows you what you will do. (Joseph, age 44)

During group analysis, community researchers stressed the dangers of drinking for those living with HIV in their community and the inevitability of HIV treatment adherence failure. Heated discussion among the community researchers broke out while reviewing participant narratives of non-adherence. One of the community researchers, during an analysis session, said "This is a big problem in the [male sex worker] community and is why some of our members are still dying—even though they have access to the drugs [ARVs]; it's not enough!" Sadly, one of community researchers passed during the study from this very fate.

3.8.2 Harm Reduction

Within the protected spaces created by HOYMAS, the first author observed how members received exposure to a wealth of information about HIV/STI vulnerability, treatment adherence, poverty, stigma and social justice and human rights. Through formal and informal discussions encouraged by HOYMAS staff, members reflected on and made sense of the myriad social and health problems facing their community, including heavy drinking. Staff attempts to engage with members around issues of problem drinking followed harm reduction logics. These logics were also reflected in the following narratives from two participants who had enrolled in HOYMAS programmes:

> Okay I am not planning on quitting but controlling the amount of alcohol I take. I used to take around 15–20 beers there, right now I have reduced to ten. Which is kind of okay to me; it is an improvement yeah. (George, 22 years)

> I tell them [my peers] that alcohol doesn't go well together with sex work. You can get a client and he takes you to the room but because you are drunk and his aim [is] to have sex with you without a condom and you don't know that. Now when you get to the room and you are so drunk, why can't he have sex with you without a condom? So, he will do it and then you might get infected. If you have HIV I and he has HIV 2, now the medicines you take for HIV I will not help you in this case. That is why I tell sex workers, if you normally drink you should reduce it. If you take five [drinks], take three. . . . That way you will be keen to use a condom, or you will know if the condom bursts and that way you can go for PEP the next day. (Patrick, 23 years)

According to the following participant narratives, receiving an HIV positive diagnosis precipitated the will to alter their drinking practices. Treated as a "wake-up call", HIV seroconversion shifted the narrative from "loss of control" to one of self-determination.

> When that happened [testing positive for HIV] I decide to quit alcohol so that I could take the medication. I saw that alcohol wasn't helping at all. You can drink and then you are stressed. The next thing you know you have to be taken to hospital. And then the medicine won't even help because when you are drunk you don't remember to take the medicine at the right time. If you don't take them at the same time every day, they will not help you. That is why I advise that they should not take alcohol if you are HIV positive. If you take your medicine and a balanced diet, you will live long, even 50 years. (Patrick, 23 years)

> Okay the moment I realized I was HIV positive and I was advised to stop from taking alcohol. I just went down, sat and made a good decision; what is better taking alcohol and dying soon or leaving alcohol and lasting for some time? Then I came to the conclusion that I need to stay because life is still sweet. I just decided that I will have to avoid alcohol so basically what I did I just avoided friends with whom I would take alcohol and created new friends with whom I would even go church with, share a cup of coffee with eventually it stopped, yeah. I just stopped friends who take alcohol and decided deeply in my heart that I and alcohol we are no longer friends. If you want to date me please buy soda, buy a cup of tea, coffee I will take, alcohol no. Yeah. (Erick, 33 years)

In many ways, these narratives about "becoming HIV positive" align with the notion of "hitting rock-bottom", an idiom that frequently appears in Alcoholics Anonymous (AA) narratives of recovery in other contexts (Weegmann & Piwowoz-Hjort, 2009).

Like the notion of hitting rock bottom, participants framed HIV seroconversion not only as a moment of fallenness and moral failure, but also as a highly generative moment in producing a self-realization that one’s life, moving forward, must somehow change (Also see Kremer et al., 2009). Importantly here, the first author observed how HOYMAS support groups for people living with HIV mediated these self-realizations and individualistic decisions around alcohol reduction and cessation through collective meaning-making exercises.

3.9 Conclusion

Participants in this study portrayed problem drinking as a tumultuous journey shaped by interlocking social problems, arriving at HIV seroconversion as the ultimate “fall”. Many viewed alcohol as beneficial and necessary to performing sex work; but the nature of the work caused some to drink to cope with stigma and stress, to tolerate sex with multiple clients, and to be able to express their erotic feelings. Thus, narratives of heavy drinking pivot on ambiguous notions of agency: alcohol enables participants to gain the courage to engage in sexual activities, while at the same time it leads to a loss of control. The danger of alcohol use, according to the narratives, lies in how it soothes social suffering while inflaming it. Male sex workers who attended HOYMAS rights-based programmes were also aware of the broader structural conditions: the criminalized status of sex work, the highly stigmatized view of homosexuality in Kenyan society, and the struggles around poverty, housing, and unemployment plaguing their community.

Given how transnationally-mediated HIV interventions proliferate ideas centring on behavioural risks and individual responsibilities, one might expect HOYMAS’ entanglements with the global health apparatus to depoliticize and mute community activist priorities. HIV prevention and treatment policy imperatives certainly do shape the web of meanings related to problem drinking expressed by our study participants. However, as a “hybrid organization” (Currier & McKay, 2017), HOYMAS merges civil rights and social justice objectives with community health aims, a reality which is reflected in the narratives of the study participants. In general, most participants did not narrate their alcohol-related problems as reducible to “poor” individual decision making, as risk-reduction counselling approaches would suggest. Instead, the advice-giving quality of their drinking narratives depicted social and health problems as shared by a wider community of male sex workers who were facing multiple oppressions. In this way, the narratives should be regarded as imbued with collective political significance. They reach outward to make broader demands on those leading global interventions to consider the exigencies surrounding alcohol use and the social and economic demands on male sex workers in Nairobi.

References

Aggleton, P., & Parker, R. (Eds.). (2014). *Men who sell sex: Global perspectives*. Routledge.

Awondo, P. (2010). The politicisation of sexuality and rise of homosexual movements in post-colonial Cameroon. *Review of African Political Economy, 37*(125), 315–328.

Baral, S., Trapence, G., Motimedi, F., Umar, E., Iipinge, S., Dausab, F., et al. (2009). HIV prevalence, risks for HIV infection, and human rights among men who have sex with men in Malawi, Namibia, and Botswana. *PLoS One, 4*(3), e4997.

Baral, S. D., Grosso, A., Holland, C., & Papworth, E. (2014). The epidemiology of HIV among men who have sex with men in countries with generalized HIV epidemics. *Current Opinion in HIV and AIDS, 9*(2), 156–167.

Coates, T., et al. (2013). *Project EXPLORE: A randomized clinical trial of the efficacy of a behavioral intervention to prevent acquisition of HIV among men who have sex with men* [Website no longer available].

Currier, A. (2012). *Out in Africa: LGBT Organizing in Namibia and South Africa*. University of Minnesota Press.

Currier, A., & McKay, T. (2017). Pursuing social justice through public health: Gender and sexual diversity activism in Malawi. *Critical African Studies, 9*(1), 71–90.

Dixon, V., Reza-Paul, S., D'Souza, F. M., O'Neil, J., O'Brien, N., & Lorway, R. (2012). Increasing access and ownership of clinical services at an HIV prevention project for sex workers in Mysore, India. *Global Public Health, 7*(7), 779–791.

Fan, E. L. (2014). HIV testing as prevention among MSM in China: The business of scaling-up. *Global Public Health, 9*(1–2), 85–97.

Geibel, S., Luchters, S., King'ola, N., Esu-Williams, E., Rinyiru, A., & Tun, W. (2008). Factors associated with self-reported unprotected anal sex among male sex workers in Mombasa, Kenya. *Sexually Transmitted Diseases, 35*(8), 746–752.

Geibel, S., King'ola, N., Temmerman, M., & Luchters, S. (2012). The impact of peer outreach on HIV knowledge and prevention behaviours of male sex workers in Mombasa, Kenya. *Sexually Transmitted Infections, 88*(5), 357–362.

Igonya, E. K. (2017). *My brother's keeper? Care, support and HIV support groups in Nairobi, Kenya*. Unpublished doctoral thesis, University of Amsterdam, the Netherlands.

Igonya, E. K., & Moyer, E. (2016). 4.1 freedom corner. In L. Manderson, E. Cartright, & A. Hardon (Eds.), *The Routledge handbook of medical anthropology* (pp. 75–80). Routledge.

Ilcan, S., & Basok, T. (2004). Community government: Voluntary agencies, social justice, and the responsibilization of citizens 1. *Citizenship Studies, 8*(2), 129–144.

Johnson, C. A., & Cameron, E. (2007). *Off the map. How HIV/AIDS programming is failing same-sex practicing people in Africa*. International Gay and Lesbian Human Rights Commission.

Kalichman, S. C., Simbayi, L. C., Cain, D., & Jooste, S. (2007). Alcohol use and sexual risks for HIV/AIDS in sub-Saharan Africa: Systematic review of empirical findings. *Prevention Science, 8*, 141–151.

Knox, J., Reddy, V., Lane, T., Lovasi, G., Hasin, D., & Sandfort, T. (2017). Determinants of hazardous drinking among black South African men who have sex with men. *Drug and Alcohol Dependence, 180*, 14–21.

Kremer, H., Ironson, G., & Kaplan, L. (2009). The fork in the road: HIV as a potential positive turning point and the role of spirituality. *AIDS Care, 21*(3), 368–377.

Lane, T., Shade, S. B., McIntyre, J., & Morin, S. F. (2008). Alcohol and sexual risk behavior among men who have sex with men in South African township communities. *AIDS and Behavior, 12*(1), S78–S85.

Lane, T., Raymond, H. F., Dladla, S., Rasethe, J., Struthers, H., McFarland, W., et al. (2011). High HIV prevalence among men who have sex with men in Soweto, South Africa: Results from the Soweto Men's Study. *AIDS and Behavior, 15*(3), 626–634.

Lorway, R. (2017). *AIDS activism, science and community across three continents*. Springer.

Lorway, R., Reza-Paul, S., & Pasha, A. (2009). On becoming a male sex worker in Mysore: Sexual subjectivity, "empowerment," and community-based HIV prevention research. *Medical Anthropology Quarterly, 23*(2), 142–160.

Lorway, R., Thompson, L., Lazarus, L., Plessis, E., Pasha, A., Mary, P., & F., et al. (2014). Going beyond the clinic: Confronting stigma and discrimination among men who have sex with men in Mysore through CBR research. *Critical Public Health, 24*(1), 73–87.

Marshall, M. (1979). *Alcoholic beverages*. University of Michigan Press.

McKinnon, L. R., Gakii, G., Juno, J. A., Izulla, P., Munyao, J., Ineri, N., et al. (2014). High HIV risk in a cohort of male sex workers from Nairobi, Kenya. *Sexually Transmitted Infections, 90*(3), 237–242.

Muraguri, N., Tun, W., Okal, J., Broz, D., Raymond, H. F., Kellogg, T., et al. (2015). HIV and STI prevalence and risk factors among male sex workers and other men who have sex with men in Nairobi, Kenya. *Journal of Acquired Immune Deficiency Syndromes, 68*(1), 91–96.

Ndjio, B. (2012). Post-colonial histories of sexuality: The political invention of a libidinal African straight. *Africa, 82*(4), 609–631.

Needle, R., Fu, J., Beyrer, C., Loo, V., Abdul-Quader, A. S., McInteyre, J. A., et al. (2012). PEPFAR's evolving HIV prevention approaches for key populations—People who inject drugs, men who have sex with men, and sex workers: Progress, challenges, and opportunities. *Journal of Acquired Immune Deficiency Syndromes, 60*, S145–S151.

Nyanzi, S. (2013). Rhetorical analysis of President Jammeh's threats to behead homosexuals in the Gambia. In S. N. Nyeck & M. Epprecht (Eds.), *Sexual diversity in Africa: Politics, theory, citizenship* (pp. 67–87). McGill-Queen's University Press.

Okal, J., Luchters, S., Geibel, S., Chersich, M. F., Lango, D., & Temmerman, M. (2009). Social context, sexual risk perceptions and stigma: HIV vulnerability among male sex workers in Mombasa, Kenya. *Culture, Health and Sexuality, 11*(8), 811–826.

Parry, C., Petersen, P., Dewing, S., Carney, T., Needle, R., Kroeger, K., et al. (2008). Rapid assessment of drug-related HIV risk among men who have sex with men in three South African cities. *Drug and Alcohol Dependence, 95*(1–2), 45–53.

Patton, C. (1990). *Inventing AIDS*. Routledge.

Purcell, D. W., Parsons, J. T., Halkitis, P. N., Mizuno, Y., & Woods, W. J. (2001). Substance use and sexual transmission risk behavior of HIV-positive men who have sex with men. *Journal of Substance Abuse, 13*(1), 185–200.

Rabinow, P., & Rose, N. (2006). Biopower today. *BioSocieties, 1*(2), 195–217.

Room, R. (1984). Alcohol and ethnography: A case of problem deflation? *Current Anthropology, 25*, 169–178.

Sandfort, T. G. M., Knox, J. R., Alcala, C., El-Bassel, N., Kuo, I., & Smith, L. R. (2017). Substance use and HIV risk among men who have sex with men in Africa: A systematic review. *Journal of Acquired Immune Deficiency Syndrome, 76*(2), 34–46.

Singer, M. (1986). Toward a political-economy of alcoholism: The missing link in the anthropology of drinking. *Social Science and Medicine, 23*(2), 113–130.

Taegtmeyer, M., Davies, A., Mwangome, M., van der Elst, E. M., Graham, S. M., Price, M. A., et al. (2013). Challenges in providing counselling to MSM in highly stigmatized contexts: Results of a qualitative study from Kenya. *PLoS One, 8*(6), e64527.

Tanser, F., de Oliveira, T., Maheu-Giroux, M., & Bärnighausen, T. (2014). Concentrated HIV sub-epidemics in generalized epidemic settings. *Current Opinion in HIV and AIDS, 9*(2), 115.

Treichler, P. A. (1999). *How to have theory in an epidemic: Cultural chronicles of AIDS*. Duke University Press.

Van der Elst, E. M., Mbogua, J., Operario, D., Mutua, G., Kuo, C., Mugo, P., Kanungi, J., Singh, S., Haberer, J., Priddy, F., & Sanders, E. J. (2013). High acceptability of HIV pre-exposure prophylaxis but challenges in adherence and use: Qualitative insights from a phase I trial of intermittent and daily PrEP in at-risk populations in Kenya. *AIDS and Behavior, 17*(6), 2162–2172.

Weegmann, M., & Piwowoz-Hjort, E. (2009). 'Naught but a story': Narratives of successful AA recovery. *Health Sociology Review, 18*(3), 273–283.

Willis, J. (2002). *Potent brews: A social history of alcohol in East Africa 1850-1999*. James Currey.

Zepeda, E., Leigh, F., Ndirangu, L., Omollo, J., & Wainaina, S. (2013). *Discussion paper: Kenya's youth employment challenge*. United Nations Development Programme.

Chapter 4
Struggles for Inclusion: Incorporating Same-Sex Practising Men into National HIV Prevention and Surveillance in African Countries, 2000–2020

Tara McKay

The global HIV policy environment changed dramatically for same-sex practising men from 2000 to 2020. These changes were especially pronounced in African countries, where research, prevention, and surveillance focused almost exclusively on heterosexual transmission for the previous 20 years. In stark contrast to the beginning of the century, by 2020, nearly all African countries identified same-sex practicing men as key populations in need of targeted HIV prevention and surveillance to control their epidemics. Drawing on a rich collection of archival, qualitative interview, and quantitative data, this chapter illuminates the global policy changes and initiatives that facilitated the recognition of the burden of HIV among same-sex practising men in African contexts, examines whether and when African countries have integrated same-sex practising men into the national HIV responses, and identifies key drivers of both inclusion and resistance to inclusion of same-sex practising men in the national HIV responses of African countries.

4.1 Creating New Global Priorities and Accountability Measures

At the beginning of the twenty-first century, staff at the Joint United Nations Programme on HIV/AIDS (UNAIDS) conducted their work in an inherent state of tension. On the one hand, the one-of-a-kind agency was tasked with promoting and achieving global consensus on HIV/AIDS policy and prevention approaches while on the other hand the organization was to respect the decisions of national policymakers.

T. McKay (✉)
Vanderbilt University, Nashville, TN, USA
e-mail: tara.mckay@vanderbilt.edu

T. Sandfort (ed.), *Male Same-sex Sexuality and HIV in Sub-Saharan Africa*, Social Aspects of HIV 7, https://doi.org/10.1007/978-3-030-73726-9_4

Like its predecessor, The Global Programme on AIDS, UNAIDS had, since its inception, sought to include gay men and other same-sex practicing men into global and national HIV policies despite opposition from member states. In the program's first operations report in 1995, UNAIDS Secretariat staff explicitly identified same-sex sexual transmission of HIV as a "major route of HIV spread" globally and insisted that "gay men living in a community where their sexual orientation is stigmatized" were a key driver of the global epidemic because of their lack of access to "life-saving information about safer sex" (UN, 1995). This was true not only in Western contexts with visible HIV epidemics among gay and bisexual men but also in most African, Asian, and Latin American, and Middle Eastern countries where little or no information on same-sex practicing men existed.

The Secretariat retained this focus on same-sex practicing men as the UNAIDS program was scaled up. In 1997, UNAIDS developed and disseminated the first technical guidelines for HIV surveillance and prevention among men who have sex with men (UNAIDS, 2000 [1997]) and repeatedly encouraged "donor and cosponsoring agencies. . .to include outreach to men who have sex with men when designing and funding national AIDS programmes" (UNAIDS, 1999, p. 40ff). Given the "inadequate or unreliable epidemiological information on HIV transmission through male-male sex. . .[and] lack of interest among donor agencies in supporting and sustaining prevention programs among men who engage in same-same sex behavior," the UNAIDS Secretariat stressed the need to "strengthen groups representing self-identified gay men, enabling them to promote HIV prevention and care programmes" throughout the world, and to review "with the aim of abolishing laws that criminalize certain sexual acts between consenting adults in private" (UNAIDS, 2000 [1997], p. 2ff). These guidelines were updated by the Secretariat in 2000 and the importance of expanding efforts to address the needs of men who have sex with men was included in the 2001 Global Strategy Framework on HIV/AIDS produced by UNAIDS (2001) and in the United Nations System Strategic Plan adopted in the same year (UN, 2001b).

However, like most other UN bodies, UNAIDS had limited power to locally enforce the policies it adopted and national AIDS programs were responsible for identifying the most relevant mode(s) of HIV transmission and the intervention strategies best suited to the local context (UN, 1995). As such, UNAIDS policy recommendations, especially those concerning same-sex practicing men, were easily dismissed or ignored by national policymakers.

The ability to hold states accountable to global HIV policy recommendations began to change in 2001. That June, almost 20 years into the epidemic, the United Nations General Assembly (UNGASS) convened a Special Session on HIV/AIDS. UNGASS was widely seen as a watershed moment in galvanizing political support for HIV prevention and treatment and establishing a global agenda. At this session, 189 United Nations (UN) member countries drafted and agreed to meet specific goals for HIV prevention and access to treatment. These goals were codified in the 2001 *Declaration of Commitment on HIV/AIDS* (UN, 2001a). The Declaration was significant in that it replaced vague commitments with specific, measurable goals and timetables for reducing HIV transmission and increasing access to care and prevention that would apply to all countries.

One of the more challenging elements for delegates to agree upon was setting universal targets for groups who were most vulnerable to HIV, deciding who constituted those groups, and reaching consensus on what should be done to protect them. While delegates unanimously supported the explicit adoption of women and children as vulnerable groups in the Declaration, some delegates excluded other more stigmatized groups, such as same-sex practising men, sex workers, and people who inject drugs from the final version of the document. To the disappointment of delegates from several member states and various nongovernment organizations (NGOs) observing the meeting, the final draft of the Declaration did not specifically identify men who have sex with men as a group in need of targeted intervention or surveillance. Nonetheless, the Declaration did encourage a "comprehensive approach to prevention" that included the expansion of human rights and prevention efforts among populations "at greatest risk of and most vulnerable to new infection as indicated by such factors as. . .sexual practices" (UN, 2001a). While this language did not explicitly identify same-sex practising men, it remained open enough to interpretation for collaborating organizations, such as the World Health Organization (WHO), to identify the development of interventions targeting men who have sex with men as a priority in their 2002 follow-up report to the UNGASS meeting (WHO, 2002).

Furthermore, by establishing universal targets for scaling up prevention and reducing infections that were endorsed by all 189 member countries, the Declaration required, for the first time, that countries submit biennial Country Progress Reports on their progress on a number of issues including surveillance infrastructure, access to prevention and HIV testing, as well as progress on enacting legal protections to prohibit discrimination towards people with HIV and vulnerable groups. The Declaration also established a standardized set of indicators so that efforts to increase the quantity and quality of services could be compared across states.

As countries collected and submitted more data from 2001 to 2008, their actions—and inactions—in relation to specific issues and population groups became much more apparent. Two years after the signing of the 2001 Declaration, the Joint United Nations Program on HIV/AIDS (UNAIDS) used the data from the first Country Progress Reports to highlight the continued absence of men who have sex with men in country-level surveillance, research and prevention activities "even when evidence points to the prominence of this mode of transmission in the epidemic" (UNAIDS, 2003, p. 5).[1] Through 2008, it was not uncommon for Country Progress Reports submitted by governments from African and Middle Eastern countries to leave blank the indicators pertaining to men who have sex with men. In other instances, countries signalled a lack of attention to this group by writing "not applicable," "not relevant," or noting in longer form that "[h]omosexuals are not

[1]See also the *Follow-up to the 2001 United Nations General Assembly Special Session on HIV/AIDS* (WHO, 2002).

among the most-at-risk groups" (Government of Rwanda, 2006, p. 41). Some governments justified their lack of inclusion of men who have sex with men through a restatement of assumed transmission dynamics. For example, the 2003 report submitted by Malawi noted that:

> The primary mode of HIV transmission in Malawi remains through unprotected heterosexual sex (90%)... Approximately 8% of transmission is believed to occur from mother to child, with annual HIV-positive births totalling more than 20,000 or about 4.2% of total births. Transmission risks due to unsafe blood products, inadequate observation of universal precautions and men having sex with men are *unknown but thought to be negligible* (2% or less). (emphasis added; Government of Malawi, 2003, p. 5)

Similarly, the 2006 progress report submitted by the Central African Republic (CAR) noted that, despite having no new surveillance data on either men who have sex with men or the general population since 1995 due to political instability, sex between men did not contribute to HIV transmission in the Republic. Rather, the report stated that, "[t]he principal mode of contamination with HIV in [the CAR] is by the hetero-sexual route...The prevention programmes (*sic*) in the CAR did not take into account the part linked to the consumption of injecting drugs, similarly those aspects linked to male homosexuality" (Government of the Central African Republic, 2005, p. 8).

To those struggling for the inclusion of same-sex practising men in global and national HIV strategies, it was clear that more funding and more research were needed to help governments 'see' the prevention and treatment needs of this population. In 2005, a stakeholder consultation on gay men and other men who have sex with men convened by UNAIDS in late 2005 concluded that:

> Across all regions, a core problem was identified as hampering the development of HIV prevention, treatment and care with men who have sex with men. Put quite simply, there is lack of funding because there is a lack of evidence; and there is a lack of evidence because there is a lack of funding. (UNAIDS, 2005b, p. 11)

To address this gap, UNAIDS collaborated with the World Health Organization to promote the strategic collection and dissemination of data on same-sex sex and HIV (UNAIDS/WHO, 2000; WHO, 2004), disseminated policy briefs (UNAIDS, 2006), established prevention guidelines for same-sex practicing men for all countries (Parker et al., 2002; UNAIDS, 2005a; WHO/UNDP, 2009), commissioned research estimating HIV infection and examining the legal obstacles to accessing prevention for same-sex practicing men in various contexts (Caceres et al., 2008a, 2008b; Anyamele et al., 2005), and funded local and regional dissemination of reports on same-sex sex and HIV (MAP, 2005).

The organization also facilitated the adoption of strategic changes in funding regulations and global policy guidelines across the UN system to encourage African governments to incorporate key populations, including men who have sex with men. In the early 2000s, a multisectoral effort was implemented across the UN system to address HIV among vulnerable populations, which included men who have sex with men and other groups. As part of this effort various UN organizations, including UNAIDS, the International Labour Organization and the United Nations

Development Programme, along with the newly-formed Global Fund to Fight AIDS, Tuberculosis and Malaria, and the World Bank collaborated to strengthen capacity to monitor the epidemic among vulnerable populations, develop and disseminate strategic information on HIV among vulnerable populations, advocate for legal protections to government officials and human rights organizations, and mobilize financial resources for supporting local programmes addressing HIV and human rights among vulnerable populations.

Throughout the early 2000s, UNAIDS also mobilized international health and development agencies to promote new funding streams for research on same-sex sex and HIV at the local, national, and regional levels. The Global Fund was a key part of this strategy. At its Sixteenth Meeting in November 2007, the Global Fund Board[2] recognized the importance of addressing gender issues in the fight against AIDS, Tuberculosis, and Malaria, placing a "particular focus on the vulnerabilities of women and girls and sexual minorities" (Global Fund, 2007a). Within a year, the Global Fund developed a parallel strategy on Sexual Orientation and Gender Identity (SOGI) and appointed new SOGI staff to increase the ability of men who have sex with men, transgender people, and female, male, and transgender sex workers to access and benefit from Global Fund grants (Global Fund, 2007b). Several internal changes were also made to ensure that proposals from civil society organizations by and for sexual and gender minorities would not be immediately rejected (Global Fund, 2007b, p. 22). Following implementation of the SOGI strategy, the participation of men who have sex with men and other groups in Global Fund awards at the country level increased (Global Fund, 2011).

In 2010, the Global Fund also established a separate stream of funding for single country and multi-country proposals from national and regional civil society groups addressing HIV among men who have sex with men, transgender people, sex workers, and injection drug users. Within this separate funding stream, 95% of proposals focused on addressing the prevention needs of men who have sex with men, transgender people and sex workers as compared with 55% of funded proposals in the general funding category (Gurkin et al., 2011).[3] The creation of this separate funding stream for key population groups may have also indirectly promoted in the prioritization of interventions focused on those that are more at risk of being infected in the general funding pool (Global Fund, 2010).

Support from the Global Fund after the 2008 SOGI strategy was implemented has significantly increased the inclusion of men who have sex with men in national HIV prevention and surveillance efforts (McKay, 2016). Figure 4.1 presents the marginal effect of support from Global Fund after 2008, as a percent of total government expenditure (lagged), on the probability of change in level of inclusion of men who have sex with men, by legal status of same-sex sex. As Global Fund support

[2]The Board is comprised of representatives from select donor and recipient countries, NGOs, and private donors.

[3]However, funded proposals in the reserve funding stream were 50% less likely to provide for treatment or care activities.

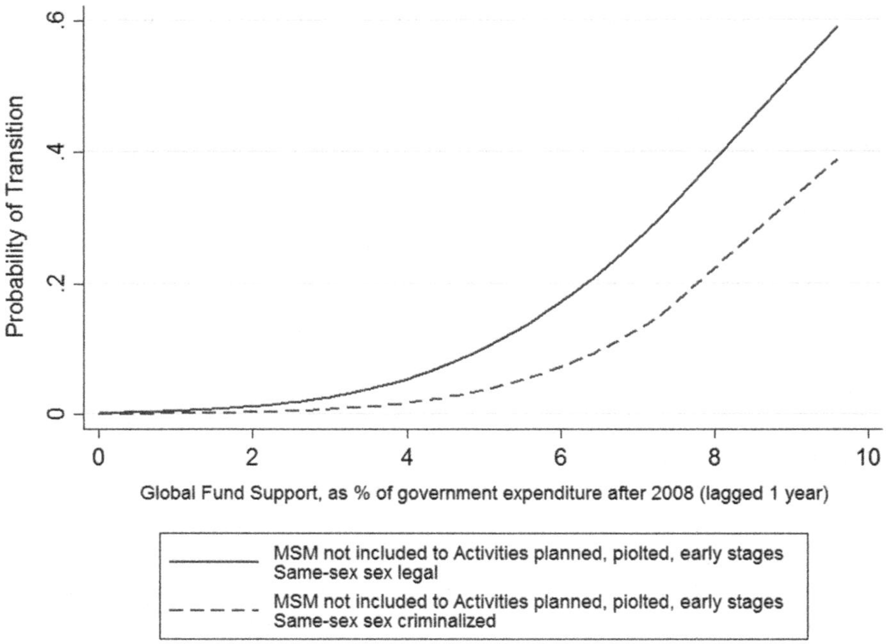

Fig. 4.1 Marginal effect of support from Global Fund after 2008, as a percent of total government expenditure (lagged), on probability of change in level of inclusion of men who have sex with men, by legal status of same-sex sex. Notes: (1) 'Activities planned' includes countries that have identified men who have sex with men as a target population, have planned or initiated pilot programs, and/or conduct prevention or surveillance activities that are highly limited in scope, geography, or internal resource commitment. (2) Regression model estimates control for a set of time varying parameters, including: national HIV prevalence (lagged), gross national income (lagged and logged), country religious composition, and year

increases, countries that have not previously acknowledged men who have sex with men are more likely to identify them as a target group for prevention and surveillance in their next Country Progress Report. This is true both in countries where same-sex sex is legal and where same-sex sex is criminalized. Among African countries, Global Fund support represents about 1–1.3% of total government expenditure from 2008 to 2016, on average, although is as high as 6–8% in some countries.

However, strategic use of funding to encourage countries to incorporate same-sex practising men appears to have some substantial limitations. By looking more closely at the level of inclusion of same-sex practising men in Country Progress Reports, the barriers to expanding programmes targeting same-sex practising men beyond the planning or pilot stages are more substantial than just naming a group on paper. Support from the Global Fund after the SOGI strategy was implemented has no effect on the probability that an African country will *expand* services targeting same-sex practising men. This suggests that the threshold for a country to initially include same-sex practicing men in national HIV planning and committing to pilot programs is likely low. However, the threshold including same-sex practicing men in

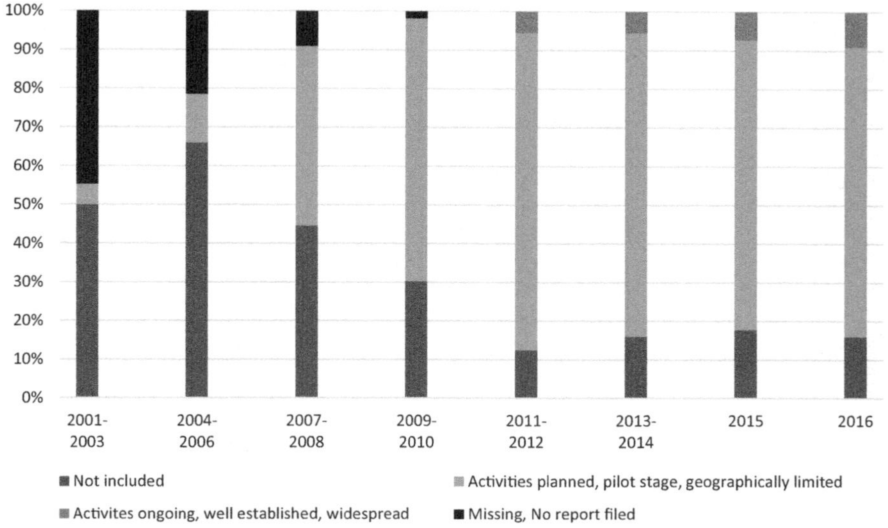

Fig. 4.2 Percent of countries on the African continent where men who have sex with men are included as a priority in HIV prevention and surveillance activities, by level of inclusion and report year. Note: 'Activities planned' includes countries that have identified men who have sex with men as a target population, have planned or initiated pilot programs, and/or conduct prevention or surveillance activities that are highly limited in scope, geography, or internal resource commitment. 'Activities widespread' includes countries that conduct prevention and surveillance among men who have sex with men in an ongoing and widespread manner. Source: UN Country Progress Reports on HIV/AIDS, 2001–2016

an expanded set of prevention programs or surveillance is much higher. In short, the value of funding incentives appears to be high for priority setting but is much lower at the implementation stage.

Due in part to the new information on same-sex practices and HIV risk and to strategic changes in how UN and multilateral agencies have sought to fund work with same-sex practising men and their communities, many countries have found it difficult to avoid[4] recognizing same-sex practising men and other LGBT populations in their national HIV strategies. Figure 4.2 presents the percentage of countries on the African continent where men who have sex with men are included as a priority in HIV prevention and surveillance activities, by level of inclusion and report year from 2001 to 2016. Compared to reports submitted by African governments in 2003 and 2006, when a majority of countries in the continent did not identify men who have sex with men as a target population, reports submitted after 2008 are significantly

[4]Interviews conducted in Malawi between 2010 and 2012 suggest that some countries likely acted strategically to gain access to new funds and/or to maintain existing relationships with funders (Currier & McKay, 2017; Angotti et al., 2019).

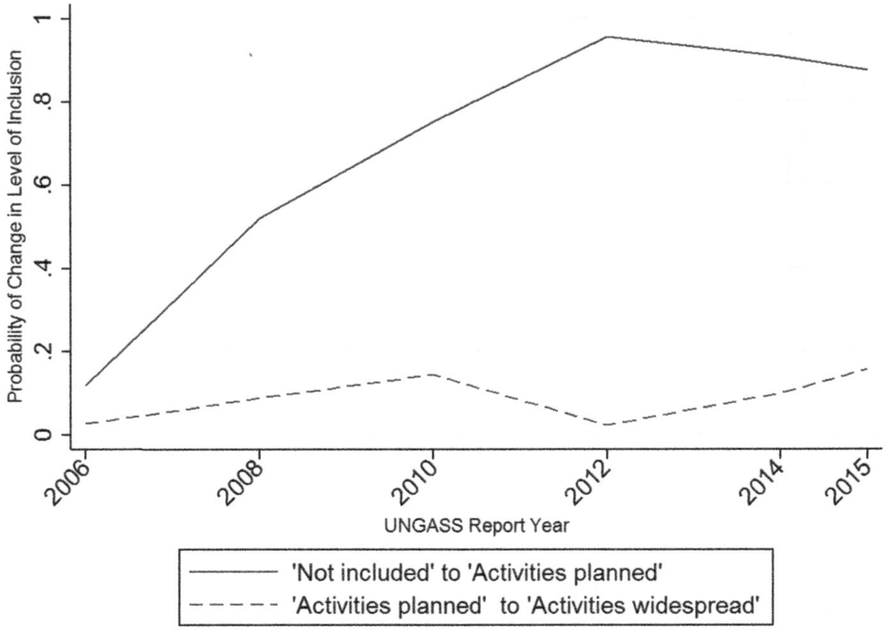

Fig. 4.3 Probability of change in level of inclusion of men who have sex with men among national HIV programs in African countries, by year and level of inclusion. Note: 'Activities planned' includes countries that have identified men who have sex with men as a target population, have planned or initiated pilot programs, and/or conduct prevention or surveillance activities that are highly limited in scope, geography, or internal resource commitment. 'Activities widespread' includes countries that conduct prevention and surveillance among men who have sex with men in an ongoing and widespread manner. Source: UNGASS Country Progress Reports, 2003–2015

more likely to identify men who have sex with men as a target group for HIV prevention and surveillance.[5]

By 2010, most African governments identified men who have sex with men as a target population in their Country Progress Reports on HIV. However, only a few countries had developed regular surveillance and widespread prevention activities targeting same-sex practicing men.

Despite an increasing probability of an African country identifying same-sex practising men as a target population for HIV prevention and surveillance up until 2012—at which point it was almost certain that any country that had not identified same-sex practising men would identify them in a subsequent report—Fig. 4.3 shows that the probability that an African country would go on to undertake regular surveillance and expand prevention activities targeting same-sex practicing men remained nearly zero up until 2015.

[5]As of 2016, very few African countries had integrated men who have sex with men into HIV prevention and surveillance in an ongoing basis.

4.2 Resistance: Contextualizing African Responses to the Epidemic and Same-Sex Sex

Although most African governments now recognize HIV transmission among same-sex practicing men, at least on paper, their initial reluctance was not entirely unexpected given more than two decades of research, prevention and planning that almost exclusively focused on heterosexual transmission in African countries. In African and other low- and middle-income countries categorized as "Pattern II" (Chin & Mann, 1988; Quinn et al., 1986), research on same-sex sex and injection drug use, the principal risk behaviours of North American and European people living with HIV, was abandoned. From 1984 to 2007, same-sex sexual behaviour was only measured in 14 of 118 (12%) epidemiological studies on AIDS in sub-Saharan Africa in which individual behavioural risk factors for contracting HIV among men were assessed (Smith et al., 2009). Instead, "African AIDS" came to be defined among epidemiological and social science researchers, doctors, policymakers and Western media through racial and cultural difference (Cerullo & Hammonds, 1988; Austin, 1989; Patton, 1999; Kitzinger & Miller, 2003 [1992]; Packard & Epstein, 1991; Treichler, 1991; Sabatier, 1988). Some early researchers suggested that African AIDS was the result of exotic cultural and sexual practices (Hrdy, 1987)[6] and "monstrous passions" (Watney, 1989) that drove Africans to have a high number and frequency of change in heterosexual partnerships (Johnson & Laga, 1988; Piot et al., 1987; Piot & Carel, 1988; Serwadda et al., 1985).[7] Across the continent, HIV prevention was integrated with existing family planning programmes (WHO, 1986; GPA, 1988; Robinson, 2017), reinforcing the invisibility of same-sex sexual transmission and having a durable effect on the priorities and practices of HIV prevention programmes on the ground. For example, research by Esacove (2016) reveals how HIV programming in Malawi promoted heteronormative and Western understandings of sex and relationships, emphasizing condom use for penile-vaginal sex, monogamy, gender equality within loving sexual partnerships, and, at its most prescriptive, abstinence in the absence of marriage. Lack of attention to other sexual behaviours has left men in countries like Malawi and Botswana without access to

---

[6]The cultural practices that Hrdy (1987) includes run the gamut from female circumcision, ritual scarification, group circumcision of boys at adolescence, to shared medical injection paraphernalia and contact with nonhuman primates.

[7]These early understandings of HIV transmission in African contexts have been durable over the course of the epidemic. Debates specifically around the role of higher levels of concurrency driving HIV transmission in African countries were revived in the mid- and late 2000s through work that revisited this earlier line of research (Epstein, 2007; Halperin & Epstein, 2004). Evidence supporting the concurrency theory is limited, however, and several empirical studies present conflicting evidence (Reniers & Watkins, 2010; see also for review Lurie & Rosenthal, 2010). See Epprecht (2008) for in-depth discussion of how constructions of African AIDS were based on entrenched understandings of African sexuality that had solidified much earlier in colonial racial projects and African nationalism.

information on how to prevent HIV transmission during sex with other men (Fay et al., 2011).

More recently, pressure from Western countries[8] and international health and development agencies to acknowledge same-sex practising men in HIV prevention and human rights work has intersected with acute concerns in some African countries around neo-colonialism, coercive Western aid practices, social and demographic change, and what it means to be African in a globalizing world (Angotti et al., 2019; Boyd, 2013; McKay & Angotti, 2016; Vorhölter, 2012; see also discussion of Zambia in Ferguson, 2006, p. 144ff). Other scholars have examined strategic political responses to same-sex practices in relation to nation building post-independence (Currier, 2010, 2012; Weiss & Bosia, 2013) and the rise of religious nationalisms (Grossman, 2015; van Klinken, 2013) as the political landscape of several countries has changed in the late twentieth century.

As a result of these intersections, politicians in a subset of African countries have pursued--and in a few cases succeeded in passing—new legislation expanding criminal penalties for same-sex practising adults. In Malawi in 2011, in the midst of tensions with Western governments on the one hand and rising opposition from Malawian civil society on the other, Parliament revived a legislative amendment to the penal code that explicitly identified sex between women as a criminal offence punishable by 5 years in prison, which Malawian President Bingu wa Mutharika quietly ratified in January 2011. In Nigeria, *The Same Sex Marriage Prohibition Act* (SSMPA), enacted in 2014, extended existing criminal penalties, which already criminalized sex between two individuals of the same sex, punishable by up to 14 years imprisonment in southern states and by death by stoning for men and lashing or imprisonment for women in Nigeria's 12 northern states that have followed Sharia law since 2000. In its final form, the 2014 SSMPA criminalized all kinds of relationships among same-sex practising Nigerians and their allies, including nonsexual relationships. Specifically, the SSMPA established new criminal penalties for entering into a same-sex marriage or civil union contract, punishable by up to 14 years imprisonment; for public displays of affection between the members of same-sex couples, punishable by up to 10 years imprisonment; and made it illegal to register, operate, or participate in gay-affiliated clubs, organizations, or meetings. The law also included criminal penalties punishable by up to

[8]Speaking at the Commonwealth Heads of Government Meeting in Perth, Australia, in 2011, Prime Minister of the United Kingdom (UK) David Cameron announced that countries receiving UK aid should "adhere to proper human rights" and that the UK would withdraw bilateral aid from countries that did not reform legislation banning homosexuality (BBC News, 2011). Two months after Cameron's announcement, the Obama Administration also decided to integrate recognition and the protection of rights of sexual minorities into foreign aid, assistance, and development programs and tasked these programs with ensuring "swift and meaningful response to serious incidents that threaten the human rights of LGBT persons abroad" (Obama, 2011, p. § 4; Clinton, 2011). During this period, US State Department officials working on the continent understood their tasks during this period to include openly promoting decriminalization of same-sex sex and providing rapid responses to negative rhetoric from national governments (Interview, 2017).

10 years imprisonment for any person or group of persons who supports, aids, or promotes gay-affiliated clubs, organizations, or activities.

Following the passage of the *SSMPA* in 2014, state and community-led violence against same-sex practicing and nongender conforming Nigerians measurably increased. A report drafted by Nigeria's lesbian, gay, bisexual and transgender (LGBT) and men who have sex with men [MSM]-identified organizations on human rights violations on the basis of real or perceived gender or sexual identity in Nigeria summarized that, during 2014 and 2015:

> [T]here is an atmosphere of apprehension within the LGBTI [lesbian, gay, bisexual, transgender, and intersex] community, with several instances of LGBTI persons being subject to arbitrary arrest by state police, religious police (in the North) and local hoodlums across the country, as well as other de-humanizing treatment. There have been a lot of negative reactions from members of the public against persons that are perceived to be LGBTI within the society. (Initiative for Equal Rights, 2015, p. 12)

In addition to state actors' use of arbitrary arrest and detention, the report identified a plurality of human rights violations, including blackmail, extortion, battery, assault, public humiliation and kidnapping, as having been perpetrated by community members throughout the country in the year following the passage of SSMPA (Initiative for Equal Rights, 2015). Additionally, organizations serving these communities report being more isolated from mainstream HIV, health, and human rights organizations.[9]

Even where efforts to extend criminal penalties were unsuccessful, however, concerns about personal safety and daily survival predominate among same-sex practising men and their communities. In Uganda, *The Anti-Homosexuality Bill*, first introduced by member of Parliament (MP) David Bahati in October of 2009, proposed to extend the maximum sentence from 14 years imprisonment to the death penalty for so-called "aggravated homosexuality"—that is, homosexual acts committed by a person who is HIV positive or is an authority figure; homosexual acts committed on minors or people with disabilities; and repeat offenders. Like Nigeria's *SSMPA*, Bahati's Bill in Uganda also imposed new criminal penalties for "aiding and abetting homosexuality" and failing to report homosexuals to the police. The original Bill also allowed Uganda to nullify any of its international and regional commitments that it deemed "contradictory to the spirit and provisions enshrined in this Act." From 2009 to 2011, Ugandan President Yoweri Museveni denounced the bill and encouraged his cabinet to rein in Bahati. The Bill was briefly tabled in 2011 when it expired without a vote before the close of the Eighth Parliament. By late 2013, however, Museveni had reversed his position. After reducing the maximum punishment from the death penalty to life imprisonment, Uganda's Ninth Parliament successfully reintroduced and passed the bill in December 2013. Museveni signed it into law in February 2014. Due to a procedural error, however, the law was ruled invalid by the Constitutional Court later the same year. The threat of the bill being reintroduced resurfaces periodically (Gettleman, 2014) and received support from

[9]Interview, 2017

Museveni as recently as October 2019 (Bhalla, 2019). Whether the original bill or a new version is ultimately passed, as Daniel Englander writes, the effects of the bill on the lives of Uganda's sexual and gender minority communities "still linger":

> In seeking to imprison or execute the half-million lesbian, gay, bisexual, and transgendered ("LGBT") people in Uganda, the Bill sparked a nationwide flare of homophobia, where citizens, politicians, and the media have branded homosexuals as "un-African," as threats to children, and as less than human. (2011, p. 1264)

Indeed, multiple human rights and news media reports since 2009 confirm that LGBT Ugandans have experienced an increase in blackmail and extortion and been targets of violence, abuse, kidnapping, imprisonment and murder even though the law was ultimately not enacted (U.S. Department of State, 2015).

Similarly, in Senegal in 2008 a group of MPs from opposition parties proposed a law increasing the fines for homosexual acts. The legislation did not ultimately pass; however, a prominent NGO called Jamra, which garnered the support of Islamic leaders in the response to AIDS in the late 1980s and 1990s, led a wide-scale campaign against homosexuality (Angotti et al., 2019; Broqua, 2016). This campaign precipitated the arrest of nine members of AIDES Senegal, all of whom were participating in an HIV prevention session at the home of director Diadji Diouf (Wal Fadjri, 2009). The men were sentenced to 8 years in prison on charges of indecent conduct and unnatural acts. They were ultimately released a few months later when the Dakar Court of Appeals overturned the sentencing on procedural grounds, a ruling widely interpreted as reflecting international pressure. Their release led to further escalation in politicized homophobia and, along with Jamra, other religious organizations began calling for the death penalty for those convicted of homosexuality.

In this context, organizations for and by same-sex practicing men in Senegal have begun to focus more on structural issues like violence against gay men and other men who have sex with men. As one self-identified LGBTI organizer explained in a 2016 interview, "We are pushing rights, confronting arbitrary arrests, extortion, and discrimination. These things are related to HIV infection and survival even though other HIV organizations probably do not see it the same way." Meanwhile, other mainstream HIV and health organizations that receive money from international health and development agencies to serve men who have sex with men have actively distanced themselves from rights-based organizing for same-sex practising Senegalese men, and, as the director of an MSM-identified organization explained, "when there are problems for us, for LGBTI in Senegal, we are alone."[10]

[10]Interview, 2016

4.3 Creating New Opportunities for Inclusion Through Research and Policy

In hostile political contexts, it has often been difficult for local organizations, researchers, and international health and development agencies to promote the explicit inclusion and recognition of same-sex practising populations for fear of state retaliation.[11] Additionally, in most African countries, there continue to be no nationally representative data on HIV prevalence, sexual behaviours, service use, or treatment access among men who have sex with men (Hakim et al., 2018), leaving activists and organizations with fewer opportunities to highlight the needs of their communities. Yet, where international agencies and researchers have been successful in building relationships with local LGBT- and MSM-identified organizations, new studies focusing on same-sex practicing men have begun to shift understandings of HIV transmission in Africa and beyond (Baral et al., 2007; Fay et al., 2011; Lane et al., 2014; Park et al., 2013; Sandfort et al., 2008).

In addition to social-behavioural and network studies, about one third of African countries have now conducted Integrated Biological and Behavioural Surveys (IBBS) or similar second-generation surveillance studies of HIV and sexual behaviour among same-sex practising men. Among African countries that have conducted an IBBS focusing on men who have sex with men, all began conducting these studies in the early 2010s or later.[12] Several additional African countries also indicate in their most recent Country Progress Reports submitted to the UN that they have planned new or continuing rounds of IBBS work among same-sex practicing men in the next 5 years, often with support from the Global Fund to Fight HIV/AIDS, Tuberculosis, and Malaria.

Importantly, however, UNAIDS, the World Health Organization (WHO), US Centers for Disease Control (CDC), and FHI360, all recommend that countries conduct IBBS surveys every 2 years in contexts with concentrated epidemics among key populations and every 3–5 years in lower-priority settings to identify emerging transmission groups and assess the impact of the response (UNAIDS/WHO, 2014; WHO et al., 2017). In at least a few African countries with concentrated and emerging epidemics among same-sex practicing men, CDC programme officers have stated in interviews that they were unable to follow this schedule with men who have sex with men due to funding limitations, the time requirements for completing just one IBBS round, and a lack of political will on the part of the US government, especially after the 2016 election.[13] At other times, local efforts were

[11]Interview, 2017

[12]African countries that have conducted IBBS/BBS focusing on men who have sex with men include Angola (2011), Botswana (2012), Burkina Faso (2017), Burundi (2014), Cameroon (2011, 2015–2016), Ghana (2011, 2017), Kenya (2010–2011), Lesotho (2013), Liberia (2013, 2018), Mali (2015), Mauritius (2010), Mozambique (2011), Namibia (2014), Nigeria (2010), Senegal (2018), South Africa (2014–2015), Togo (2017), and Uganda (2012–2013).

[13]Interview, 2017

stymied by low prioritization among national governments. These sentiments from programme officers echo findings from broader research that national governments prioritize general population surveys over key populations and service provision over data despite awareness of likely concentrated epidemics (Hakim et al., 2018).

4.4 Increasing Space for Civil Society Organizations?

As data and funding have shifted ideas about where to prioritize prevention and surveillance efforts, organizations by and for same-sex practising men and, in some African countries, broader LGBT-identified organizations, are increasingly invited to planning meetings with other civil society organizations and ministry of health officials. As a representative from one international health agency explained in an interview concerning inclusion of same-sex practising men in Mozambique in 2017:

> There is a lot of institutional space for [the country's sole LGBT-identified organization] Lambda within the Ministry of Health, especially around HIV. They are invited, consulted, and listened to. . .The Ministry of Health does not shy away from working with them. And among civil society organizations, they are well respected and asked to represent other organizations and speak for all key population groups.

The expansion of institutional space for Lambda is reflected in Mozambique's Country Progress Reports. Prior to the 2016 Country Progress Report (República de Moçambique, 2016), government officials did not identify men who have sex with men as a target population in HIV prevention, planning or surveillance activities. In 2015, the government moved to remove the country's anti-sodomy provision from the Penal Code, which, at the time, was interpreted as a carryover from Portuguese colonial rule and not reflective of Mozambican culture. Mozambique's 2016 Country Progress Report submitted to UNAIDS immediately following decriminalization identifies men who have sex with men as a target group and details current efforts and government collaboration with Lambda to reach same-sex practising men with HIV prevention (República de Moçambique, 2016).[14]

While international health and development agencies may have been supportive of Lambda's involvement in HIV planning,[15] the organization's relationship with government institutions beyond the Ministry of Health has remained tenuous. Lambda continues to face challenges from the Ministry of Justice and was not allowed to formally register as a civil society organization for almost a decade. Although the organization received a favourable court ruling on this matter in 2017, the inability to register the organization for several years has had specific

[14]Notably, Lambda's efforts here date back to the mid-2000s but were not included in official information before 2016.

[15]Interview, 2017

consequences for funding, since it was prohibited the from opening a bank account, making it more difficult to pay staff.[16]

The uneven recognition of Lambda by government institutions affects how some within the organization think about priorities. As one Lambda staff member we interviewed explained, "Our rights stop at health. We want more than HIV. We want more than to be considered just a risk group."[17] Additionally, multiple observers have commented on the closing institutional space for civil society organizations in Mozambique. "We're being squeezed by the government," an organizer working in gender and human rights explained. "If they don't like something you are saying, they will just kill you."[18] Closing institutional space is a problem not just for LGBT- and MSM-identified organizations. In multiple countries, including Mozambique, Malawi, Nigeria, and Uganda, bills have been proposed or passed that have sought to regulate NGOs' relationships with international funders, the kind of work they engage in, and which kinds of organizations are able to officially register with the government.

In Nigeria, the International Centre for Advocacy on Rights to Health (ICARH) has forged strong relationships with funders and some government officials, especially in relation to HIV and health. In the late 2000s, ICARH founded a standalone clinic for key populations to provide an alternative to mainstream health services which many of their same-sex practising constituents found discriminatory or of low quality.[19] The organization and its clinic are well-known and attract same-sex practising men looking for HIV testing and treatment from across the country's Northern region.[20]

Because ICARH works in a criminalized context, and one that has become increasingly hostile since the passage of the *Same Sex Marriage Prohibition Act* in 2014, the organization leverages the strong belief in Nigeria that citizens have the right to health care. Doing so, it has created a space for work with LGBT-identified and other same-sex practicing populations. Using the language of health helps ICARH get around controversial issues of sexuality and morality, explained one member of the leadership. "Otherwise," he continued, "people say, 'you're promoting being gay,' which is illegal. So, instead we provide health care for everyone."[21] As in other African countries (Currier & Cruz, 2014; Currier & McKay, 2017), working in a highly politicized and criminalized context has pushed ICARH to expand the work that it does. The organization now employs a legal team to challenge aspects of the *Same Sex Marriage Prohibition Act* and defend Nigerians who are arrested for their sexual activity or gender identity. "The only way forward

[16]Interview, 2017

[17]Interview, 2017

[18]Interview, 2017

[19]Interview, 2017

[20]Interview, 2017

[21]Interview, 2017

is through dialogue with stakeholders and policymakers," concluded a member of the leadership.

4.5 New Challenges

As countries have become more attentive to same-sex sexualities, new challenges have emerged. Conversations with LGBT- and MSM-identified groups and organizations, international health and development agencies, and national government officials identified new challenges relating to including and engaging the perspectives of same-sex practising communities. Among the top challenges mentioned were issues specific to the creation of a truly inclusive community and engagement across sectors. These issues are complex and multifaceted. In several countries, for example, it has been difficult for community groups to engage older and wealthier same-sex practising men in HIV prevention and community mobilization. In South Africa, researchers estimate that about 30% of men who have sex with men are not engaged or do not want to be reached by an HIV or men's health programme and an additional 20% seek care from private providers (McIntyre, 2018). In Mozambique, these issues intersect with race/ethnicity, as older Portuguese men are less likely to be involved in grassroots HIV prevention, often led by younger and Black African staff and community members.[22] Organizers described this issue as problematic for creating an engaged, inclusive community. National programme staff at international health and development agencies also identified this as a problem because it has left them unable to reach all men who have sex with men with HIV prevention and surveillance programmes.[23]

In response to these challenges to, LGBT- and MSM-identified organizations have begun engaging in various novel activities to change policy and public opinion. These include everything from the development of short television and radio programmes featuring same-sex attracted characters; to holding training with the police, religious leaders and media organisations; to legal activism. LGBT- and MSM-identified organizations often do not have funding to conduct this work and engage in it on their own. Increasingly, both grassroots organizations and international agencies alike recognize that HIV is not the only issue affecting gender and sexual minorities, or even the only *health* issue faced by same-sex practising individuals and communities. However, international health and development agencies frequently feel their hands are tied. As a supervisor of a "key populations" programme for USAID explained:

> We understand that there are other issues that these organizations may want to address besides health. We try to help them get to those through relationships with other organizations and conversations with other ministries, like Justice and Education, but we are funded

[22]Interview, 2017

[23]Interview, 2017

> to do health. We are a health department and Key Populations is mostly if not all HIV money. We have to work within those constraints.

As a result of tight funding, LGBT- and MSM-identified organizations across Africa struggle to find funding for general budget support and human rights work that is not directly connected to HIV prevention, testing, or treatment. And while many groups have been able to successfully engage with their country's National AIDS Commission or Ministry of Health, the same cannot be said for other ministries, especially ministries of Justice, in most countries.

Moreover, the prioritization of work with men who have sex with men has led to some fragmentation within LGBT movements in several countries, where same-sex practising women in particular feel excluded from "the boys club",[24] and contexts where LGBT rights issues are frequently understood as separate from other human rights concerns.[25] Some mainstream HIV organizations also struggle with changes in funding priorities. At least a few prominent organizations resent the fact that they now must compete with LGBT- and MSM-identified organizations for funding and are forced to include them in their prevention work. As the director of one large HIV organization in Nigeria explained:

> Key populations are too powerful. They go directly to Geneva and then Geneva tells us we have to include them here, too. They tell us we must include them. We do work with key populations indirectly, but not directly. It is very difficult to work with these groups because politically it is very problematic. People can go to jail for 12 to 15 years.

While this sentiment may reflect personal bias against LGBT- and MSM-identified communities in addition to organizational concerns, points of fracture across civil society and the difficulty of engaging a broad coalition across sectors poses serious, ongoing problems for LGBT- and MSM-identified groups working in HIV prevention, limiting the effectiveness, resilience, and adaptability of LGBT and MSM community organizations across the continent.

4.6 Conclusion

By 2020, same-sex practising men and their communities were included in HIV policy and programmes in ways that were unthinkable 20 years ago. Nowhere is this truer than in African countries. Nearly all African countries now identify men who have sex with men as a population in need of targeted HIV prevention and surveillance in their Country Progress Reports submitted to the United Nations. The wide inclusion of same-sex practising men was never inevitable and reflects massive, strategic undertakings to change the policy and funding landscapes at the global, national, and local levels. These changes ultimately increased accountability among

---

[24] Interview, 2017

[25] Interview, 2017

UN member states, encouraged the inclusion of same-sex practising men in HIV prevention and surveillance, and supported the mobilization of same-sex sexualities in indifferent and hostile political contexts.

Despite this progress, substantial challenges remain. The attention of local and international health and development organizations on HIV among same-sex practising men has drawn backlash from political and religious elites in several African countries. Additionally, several African countries continue to have little or no epidemiological or surveillance data tracking HIV among same-sex practising men. In some Country Progress Reports, HIV prevalence or risk behaviour data on men who have sex with men are more than 5 years out of date, are only presented for men in the capital city, or are only presented for men in major cities. These data gaps make it difficult to track—and prevent—new infections; they also limit the ability of local and international groups to effectively advocate for the prioritization of key population groups like same-sex practising men in national funding allocations.

On the ground, institutional space for LGBT- and MSM-identified groups and organizations has increased in several African countries over the past 20 years. Members of these groups and organizations are frequently invited to events, consulted in planning processes, and, in many cases, consulted by officials representing the Ministry of Health and international health and development agencies. LGBT- and MSM-identified groups and organizations remain central to the global response to HIV. Within this space, interventions by and for men who have sex with men have emerged and continue to be advanced by local and globalized discourses that support a right to health for all citizens.

Yet, while these discourses have been effective in promoting work to support LGBT-identified and other community members, the limits of a rights to health framework are quickly coming into focus for organizations and international agencies working on the continent. Research suggests that, on the ground, LGBT- and MSM-identified organizations experience these discourses—and the funding requirements that accompany them—as severely limiting. Meanwhile, some LGBT- and MSM-identified organizations have been rejected by mainstream health and rights organizations struggling to adapt to changes in the international funding landscape while others have had to contend with more general attacks on civil society by political elites.

Finally, although many African countries acknowledge men who have sex with men as a key target population on paper, very few have taken the next step of purposeful engagement in prevention and treatment activities. Key features of the global system that previously supported the inclusion of sexual and gender minorities may now also be driving backlash (Velasco, 2019), making the goal of meaningful inclusion even harder to achieve. However, a country's acknowledgement of same-sex practising men provides an important point of leverage for targeted advocacy from above and below to ensure that countries take the next step in ensuring the meaningful and widespread inclusion in HIV prevention and treatment programming.

References

Angotti, N., McKay, T., & Robinson, R. S. (2019). HIV interventions, LGBT visibility, and anti-gay backlash in African countries. *Sociology of Development, 5*(1), 71–90.

Anyamele, C., Lwabaayi, R., Nguyen, T.-V., & Binswanger, H. (2005). Sexual minorities, violence and AIDS in Africa. *The World Bank Africa Region Working Paper Series, 84*, 1–35.

Austin, S. B. (1989). AIDS and Africa: United States media and racist fantasy. *Cultural Critique, 14*, 129–152.

Baral, S., Sifakis, F., Cleghorn, F., & Beyrer, C. (2007). Elevated risk for HIV infection among men who have sex with men in low- and middle-income countries 2000–2006: A systematic review. *PLoS Medicine, 4*, 1901–1911.

BBC News. (2011). Cameron threat to dock some UK aid to anti-gay nations. *BBC News*. Retrieved October 9, 2012, from http://www.bbc.co.uk/news/uk-15511081

Bhalla, N. (2019, October 10). Uganda plans bill imposing death penalty for gay sex. *Reuters*.

Boyd, L. (2013). The problem with freedom: Homosexuality and human rights in Uganda. *Anthropological Quarterly, 86*(3), 697–724.

Broqua, C. (2016). Islamic movements against homosexuality in Senegal. In A. van Klinken & E. Chitando (Eds.), *Public religion and the politics of homosexuality in Africa* (pp. 163–179). Routledge.

Caceres, C. F., Konda, K., Segura, E. R., & Lyerla, R. (2008a). Epidemiology of male same-sex behaviour and associated sexual health indicators in low- and middle-income countries: 2003–2007 estimates. *Sexually Transmitted Infections, 84*(suppl 1), i49–i56.

Caceres, C. F., Pecheny, M., Frasca, T., Rios, R. R., & Pocahy, F. (2008b). *Report to the joint united review of legal frameworks and the situation of human rights related to sexual diversity in low and middle income countriesations programme on HIV/AIDS*. Joint United Nations Programme on HIV/AIDS.

Cerullo, M., & Hammonds, E. (1988). AIDS in Africa: The Western imagination and the dark continent. *Radical America, 21*, 21.

Chin, J., & Mann, J. M. (1988). The global patterns and prevalence of AIDS and HIV infection. *AIDS, 2*(suppl 1), s247–s252.

Clinton, H. R. (2011, December 6). *Remarks in recognition of International Human Rights Day*. Retrieved October 9, 2012, from U.S. Department of State: http://www.state.gov/secretary/rm/2011/12/178368.htm

Currier, A. (2010). Political homophobia in postcolonial Namibia. *Gender and Society, 24*(1), 110–129.

Currier, A. (2012). *Out: LGBT organizing in Namibia and South Africa*. University of Minnesota Press.

Currier, A., & Cruz, J. M. (2014). Civil society and sexual struggles in Africa. In E. Obadare (Ed.), *The handbook of civil society in Africa* (pp. 337–360). Springer.

Currier, A., & McKay, T. (2017). Pursuing social justice through public health: Gender and sexual diversity activism in Malawi. *Critical African Studies, 9*(1), 71–90.

Englander, D. (2011). Protecting the human rights of LGBT people in Uganda in the wake of Uganda's "Anti Homosexuality Bill, 2009". *Emory International Law Review, 25*, 1263–1316.

Epprecht, M. (2008). *Heterosexual Africa? The history of an idea from the age of exploration to the age of AIDS*. Ohio University Press.

Epstein, H. (2007). *The invisible cure: Why we are losing the fight against AIDS in Africa*. Picador.

Esacove, A. (2016). *Modernizing sexuality: U.S. HIV prevention in Sub-Saharan Africa*. Oxford University Press.

Fay, H., Baral, S. D., Trapence, G., Motimed, F., Umar, E., Iipinge, S., et al. (2011). Stigma, health care access, and HIV knowledge among men who have sex with men in Malawi, Namibia, and Botswana. *AIDS and Behavior, 15*(6), 1088–1097.

Ferguson, J. (2006). *Global shadows: Africa in the neoliberal world order*. Duke University Press.

Gettleman, J. (2014 йил 1–August). Uganda anti-gay law struck down by court. *New York Times*.

Global Fund. (2007a). *Sixteenth board meeting, 12–13 November*. The Global Fund to Fight AIDS, Tuberculosis and Malaria.

Global Fund. (2007b). *The global fund strategy in relation to sexual orientation and gender identity*. The Global Fund to Fight HIV/AIDS, Tuberculosis and Malaria.

Global Fund. (2010). *Report of the technical review panel and the secretariat on round 10 proposals*. Global Fund to Fight HIV/AIDS, Tuberculosis and Malaria, Technical Review Panel.

Global Fund. (2011). *Analysis of rounds 8, 9 and 10 Global Fund HIV proposals in relation to men who have sex with men, transgender people and sex workers*. Global Fund to Fight HIV/AIDS, Tuberculosis and Malaria.

Government of Malawi. (2003). *Follow up to the declaration of commitment on HIV/AIDS (UNGASS): Country report for Malawi, January–December 2002*. Government of Malawi.

Government of Rwanda. (2006). *Rwanda: Follow-up to the declaration of committment on HIV/AIDS (UNGASS)*. Government of Rwanda.

Government of the Central African Republic. (2005). *Central African Republic: UNGASS report 2003–2005*. Government of the Central African Republic.

GPA. (1988). *Progress report number 4*. The World Health Organization, Global Programme on AIDS.

Grossman, G. (2015). Renewalist christianity and the political saliency of LGBTs: Theory and evidence from Sub-Saharan Africa. *Journal of Politics, 77*(2), 337–351.

Gurkin, A., Graham, A., & Seale, A. (2011). *Analysis of Rounds 8, 9 and 10 Global Fund HIV proposals in relation to men who have sex with men, transgender people and sex workers*. Global Fund to Fight HIV/AIDS, Tuberculosis and Malaria.

Hakim, A. J., MacDonald, V., Hladik, W., Zhao, J., Burnett, J., Sabin, K., et al. (2018). Gaps and opportunities: Measuring the key population cascadethrough surveys and services to guide the HIV response. *Journal of the International AIDS Society, 21*(s5), e25119.

Halperin, D. T., & Epstein, H. (2004). Concurrent sexual partnerships help to explain Africa's high HIV prevalence: Implications for prevention. *The Lancet, 364*, 4–6.

Hrdy, D. B. (1987). Cultural practices contributing to the transmission of human immunodeficiency virus in Africa. *Reviews of Infectious Diseases, 9*(6), 1109–1119.

Initiative for Equal Rights. (2015). *Report on human rights violations based on real of perceived sexual orientation and gender identity in Nigeria*. Initiative for Equal Rights.

Johnson, A. M., & Laga, M. (1988). Heterosexual transmission of HIV. *AIDS, 2*(suppl 1), s49–s56.

Kitzinger, J., & Miller, D. (2003 [1992]). 'African AIDS': The media and audience beliefs. In P. Aggleton & P. M. DAvies (Eds.), *AIDS: Rights, risk and reason* (pp. 28–52). RoutledgeFalmer.

Lane, T., Osmand, T., Marr, A., Shade, S. B., Dunkle, K., Sandfort, T., et al. (2014). The Mpumalanga Men's Study (MPMS): Results of a baseline biological and behavioral HIV surveillance survey in two MSM communities in South Africa. *PLoS One, 9*(11), e111063–e111063.

Lurie, M. N., & Rosenthal, S. (2010). Concurrent partnerships as a driver of the HIV epidemic in sub-Saharan Africa? The evidence is limited. *AIDS and Behavior, 14*(1), 17–24.

MAP. (2005). *Male-male sex and AHIV/AIDS in Asia*. The Monitoring the AIDS Pandemic Network.

McIntyre, J. (2018). *The HIV epidemic in MSM in South Africa*. Microbicide trials network regional meeting. Cape Town.

McKay, T. (2016). From Marginal to marginalised: The inclusion of men who have sex with men in global and national AIDS programmes and policy. *Global Public Health, 11*(7–8), 902–922.

McKay, T., & Angotti, N. (2016). Ready rhetorics: Political homophobia and activist discourses in Malawi, Nigeria, and Uganda. *Qualitative Sociology, 39*(4), 397–420.

Obama, B. (2011, December 6). *Presidential memorandum—International initiatives to advance the human rights of lesbian, gay, bisexual, and transgender persons*. Retrieved October 9, 2012, from The White House, Office of the Press Secretary: http://www.whitehouse.gov/the-press-office/2011/12/06/presidential-memorandum-international-initiatives-advance-human-rights-l

Packard, R. M., & Epstein, P. (1991). Medical research on AIDS in Africa: A historical perspective. In E. Fee & D. M. Fox (Eds.), *AIDS: The making of a chronic disease* (pp. 346–376). University of California Press.

Park, J. N., Papworth, E., Kassegne, S., Moukam, L., Billong, S. C., Macauley, I., et al. (2013). HIV prevalence and factors associated with HIV infection among men who have sex with men in Cameroon. *Journal of the International AIDS Society, 16*(4S3), 18752.

Parker, R., Caceres, C. F., Khan, S., & Aggleton, P. (2002). Reaching men who have sex with men. In P. R. Lamptey & H. D. Gayle (Eds.), *HIV/AIDS prevention in resource-constrained settings: A handbook for the design and management of programs* (pp. 259–280). Family Health International.

Patton, C. (1999). Inventing 'African AIDS'. In P. Aggleton & R. Parker (Eds.), *Culture, society and sexuality: A reader* (1st ed., pp. 387–404). University College London Press.

Piot, P., & Carel, M. (1988). Epidemiological and sociological aspects of HIV-infection in developing countries. *British Medical Bulletin, 44*, 68–88.

Piot, P., Kreiss, J. K., Ndinya-Achola, J. O., Ngugi, E. N., Simonsen, J. N., Cameron, D. W., et al. (1987). Heterosexual transmission of HIV. *AIDS, 1*, 199–206.

Quinn, T. C., Mann, J. M., Curran, J. W., & Piot, P. (1986). AIDS in Africa: An epidemiologic paradigm. *Science, 234*(4779), 955–963.

Reniers, G., & Watkins, S. C. (2010). Polygyny and the spread of HIV in Sub Saharan Africa: A case of benign concurrency. *AIDS, 24*(2), 299–307.

República de Moçambique. (2016). *Resposta Global à SIDA: Relatório do Progresso, 2016: MOÇAMBIQUE*. Conselho Nacional de Combate ao SIDA.

Robinson, R. S. (2017). *Intimate interventions in global health: Family planning and HIV prevention in Sub-Saharan Africa*. Cambridge University Press.

Sabatier, R. (1988). *Blaming others: Prejudice, race and worldwide AIDS*. PANOS Institute.

Sandfort, T. G., Nel, J., Rich, E., Reddy, V., & Yi, H. (2008). HIV testing and self-reported HIV status in South African men who have sex with men: Results from a community-based survey. *Sexually Transmitted Infections, 84*(6), 425–429.

Serwadda, D., Swankambo, N. K., Carswell, J. W., Bayley, A. C., Tedder, R. S., Weiss, R. A., et al. (1985). Slim disease: A new disease in Uganda and its assoctiation with HTLV-III infection. *The Lancet, 326*(8460), 849–852.

Smith, A., Tapsoba, P., Peshu, N., Sanders, E. J., & Jaffe, H. W. (2009). Men who have sex with men and HIV/AIDS in sub-Saharan Africa. *The Lancet, 374*, 416–422.

Treichler, P. (1991). AIDS and HIV infection in the third world: A first world chronicle. In E. Fee & D. M. Fox (Eds.), *AIDS: The making of a chronic disease* (pp. 377–401). University of California Press.

U.S. Department of State. (2015). *Uganda 2015 human rights report*. Government of the United States of America.

UN. (1995). *Report of the Committee of Co-sponsoring Organizations of the Joint and Co-sponsored United Nations programme on HIV/AIDS (E/1995/71)*. United Nations, Economic and Social Council.

UN. (2001a). *Declaration of commitment on HIV/AIDS*. United Nations General Assemblty.

UN. (2001b). *United Nations system strategic plan for HIV/AIDS for 2001–2005*. United Nations.

UNAIDS. (1999). *The UNAIDS report*. Joint United Nations Programme on HIV/AIDS.

UNAIDS. (2000 [1997]). *AIDS and men who have sex with men: UNAIDS technical update*. Joint United Nations Programme on HIV/AIDS.

UNAIDS. (2001). *The global strategy framework on HIV/AIDS*. The Joint United Nations Programme on HIV/AIDS.

UNAIDS. (2003). *AIDS epidemic update: December 2003*. The Joint United Nations Programme on HIV/AIDS and the World Health Organization.

UNAIDS. (2005a). *Intensifying HIV prevention*. Policy position paper, Joint United Nations Programme on HIV/AIDS, Geneva.

UNAIDS. (2005b). *Men who have sex with men, HIV prevention and care: Report of a UNAIDS stakeholder consultation.* Joint United Nations Programme on HIV/AIDS (UNAIDS). Retrieved March 5, 2011, from UNAIDS.
UNAIDS. (2006). *HIV and sex between men: Policy brief.* Retrieved March 5, 2011, from UNAIDS: http://www.unaids.org/en/media/unaids/contentassets/dataimport/publications/irc-pub07/jc1269-policybrief-msm_en.pdf
UNAIDS/WHO. (2000). *Guidelines for second generation HIV surveillance.* Joint United Nations Programme on HIV/AIDS and the World Health Organization, Working Group on Global HIV/AIDS and STI Surveillance.
UNAIDS/WHO. (2014). *Guidelines for second generation HIV surveillance: An update: Know your epidemic.* UNAIDS/WHO Working Group on Global HIV/AIDS and STI Surveillance. World Health Organization.
van Klinken, A. (2013). Gay rights, the devil and the end times: Public religion and the enchantment of the homosexuality debate in Zambia. *Religion, 43*(4), 519–540.
Velasco, K. (2019). A growing queer divide: The divergence between transnational advocacy networks and foreign aid in diffusing LGBT policies. *International Studies Quarterly, 64*(1), 120–132.
Vorhölter, J. (2012). Negotiating social change: Ugandan discourses on Westernization and neo-colonialism as forms of social critique. *Journal of Modern African Studies, 50*(2), 283–307.
Wal Fadjri. (2009, January 19). Pour obtenir la libération des neuf homosexuels condamnés au Sénégal: Le maire de Paris écrit aux autorités sénégalaises [To obtain release of the nine homosexuals condemned in Senegal, mayor of Paris writes to Senegalese authorities. *Wal Fadjri (Senegal).*
Watney, S. (1989). Missionary positions: AIDS, 'Africa', and race. *Critical Quarterly, 31*(3), 45–62.
Weiss, M. L., & Bosia, M. J. (2013). *Global homophobia: States, movements, and the politics of repression.* University of Illinois Press.
WHO. (1986, November 11–13). *Report of the first regional conference on AIDS in Africa.* World Health Organization, Special Program on AIDS, Brazzaville.
WHO. (2002). *Follow up on the United Nations General Assembly special session on HIV/AIDS: Work of WHO.* World Health Organization, Department of HIV/AIDS.
WHO. (2004). *Rapid assessment and response adaptation guide on HIV and men who have sex with men.* World Health Organization, Department of HIV/AIDS.
WHO, CDC, UNAIDS, FHI 360. (2017). *Biobehavioral survey guidelines for popula-tions at risk for HIV.* World Health Organization.
WHO/UNDP. (2009). *Prevention and treatment of HIV and other sexually transmitted infections among men who have sex with men and transgender populations: Report of a technical consultation, 15–17 September 2008.* Meeting report. World Health Organization and the United Nations Development Programme, Geneva.

Chapter 5
Hardship, Public Health, *Heshima*, Lube and Problem Trees: Forces Shaping Grassroots Organizing Against HIV Among Same-Sex Attracted Men in Dar es Salaam

Kåre Moen, Elia John Mmbaga, Alexander Mwijage Ishungisa, and Melkizedeck Thomas Leshabari

This chapter aims to identify the role of human and non-human actors in the emergence and expansion of grassroots organizing for HIV prevention among same-sex attracted men in Dar es Salaam, Tanzania. It draws on ethnographic fieldwork, including long-term participant observation in community-based groups and interviews with grassroots activists, community members, health care workers, community leaders, policy makers and planners involved in programming focusing on same-sex attracted men and their HIV and health-related challenges. It discusses ten actors influential in grassroots organizing: (1) hardship, (2) HIV, (3) the field of public health, (4) men's sexual practices, (5) the concept of *heshima* (dignity, honour, respect, and courtesy) (6) the concept of key populations, (7) sexual lubricants, (8) religion, (9) funding agencies, and (10) money. It describes how grassroots actors in Dar es Salaam have been able to adapt and multiply their community-based work in spite of significant challenges. By drawing on the values inherent in *heshima*, they have found allies in unexpected places (e.g., in the church), practised reasoned subversion (e.g., by establishing alternative lube supply lines), and created widespread community awareness and action through dialogical education.

K. Moen (✉) · E. J. Mmbaga
Faculty of Medicine, Department of Community Medicine and Global Health, Institute of Heath and Society, University of Oslo, Oslo, Norway
e-mail: kare.moen@medisin.uio.no; elia.mmbaga@medisin.uio.no

A. M. Ishungisa · M. T. Leshabari
Muhimbili University of Health and Allied Sciences, Dar es Salaam, Tanzania

T. Sandfort (ed.), *Male Same-sex Sexuality and HIV in Sub-Saharan Africa*, Social Aspects of HIV 7, https://doi.org/10.1007/978-3-030-73726-9_5

5.1 Introduction

Based on long-term research in Dar es Salaam, this chapter aims to identify human and non-human actors and their role in the emergence and expansion of grassroots organising for HIV prevention among same-sex attracted men in Tanzania's largest city over the past decade. Who and what are these actors, and how have they shaped grassroots efforts to respond to the challenges of HIV?

Since the beginning of the HIV pandemic, community efforts have played a key role in shaping the overall response (Collins et al., 2016; Kameni et al., 2019; Stahlman et al., 2016). UNAIDS (2016) finds that community action has "proven critical in overcoming many of the major challenges in the AIDS response, including reaching people most affected by HIV with life-changing HIV services, and providing support for adherence to treatment and other essential health services". Evaluations of community responses in eight different countries concluded that community action can substantially improve knowledge about HIV, lead to better access to and use of HIV services, and decrease HIV incidence (Rodriguez-García et al., 2013). Civil society engagement has also played a critical role in advocating for critical resources and promoting human rights issues (UNAIDS & Stop AIDS Alliance, 2015), and UNAIDS (2016) predicts that civil society action is "essential" to ending the HIV epidemic among key populations.

Dar es Salaam, which has a population of around five million (National Bureau of Statistics, 2012), is home to a large and diverse community of same-sex attracted men. Over the past decade, considerable grassroots organising for HIV prevention has emerged within this community. While a couple of community groups have a longer history, most of the organising began after 2010. At least a dozen groups have engaged in activities to provide community members with information and education, condoms and lubricants, counselling and HIV testing, and linkage to medical care. Community groups have also contributed significantly to the work of others, including carrying out fieldwork for research projects and serving as discussion and/or implementation partners for HIV prevention programming. Our aim in this chapter is to describe and analyse the conditions that have shaped the work of these community-based groups, drawing inspiration from Latour's theorization of action.

Rather than conceiving of actors as "pure and unproblematic source[s] of action", Latour (2007, p. 46) argues that we conceive of them as entities that are "*made to act*" (ibid.). It is typically not one, but rather a plenitude of agents that bring about action, and they may be human as well as non-human. Let us offer a simple example to illustrate these points. If we wanted to understand how the authors came to write the chapters of this book, we might want to identify the range of entities that enabled them to type up their manuscripts. Among the many possible agents we might have to consider would be humans, including teachers who taught the authors to write; family members who took care of chores at home so that they would have time to work on their manuscripts; and the book editors who kept them focused on the task by regularly reminding them of manuscript submission deadlines. In addition, a range of *things* probably also played a role. While objects may not have the same agency as humans in all respects, objects and other non-humans are nonetheless entities that may do things. Among possible non-human actions could be to "authorize, allow, afford, encourage, permit, suggest, influence, block, render possible, forbid, and so on" (ibid., p. 72). When typing up this chapter, several tables and chairs enabled us to work on the manuscript, while electricity from the Tanzania Electric Supply Company kept our offices lit and our computers running and thus helped render our writing possible.

In short, Latour defines an actor as anyone or anything that is made to act by others in such a way that it comes to modify "a state of affairs by making a difference" (ibid., p. 71). To identify an actor, the question we should ask is: "Does it make a difference in the course of some other agent's action or not?" (ibid., p. 71). This concept inspires the questions we try to answer in this chapter: who and what were the actors, broadly understood, that have contributed to shape community-based organising for HIV prevention among same-sex attracted men in Dar es Salaam over the past decade? What difference have they made? How have they contributed to bring about, slow down, speed up, hinder, strengthen and shape such activism, and how have these actors mediated between same-sex attracted men, on the one hand, and HIV and its potential consequences, on the other?

5.2 Methods

This chapter draws on ethnographic fieldwork carried out by the first author in Dar es Salaam between 2014 and 2019. The research entailed long-term participant observation in community-based groups and interviews with grassroots activists, community members, health care workers, community leaders, policy makers and planners, and academics who were involved in research focusing on same-sex attracted men and their HIV and health-related challenges.

The chapter also draws on the wider, long-term research engagement that all of the authors have had with HIV-related challenges among same-sex attracted men in Tanzania. Together, we have carried out both qualitative and quantitative research with same-sex attracted men in Dar es Salaam and other Tanzanian cities since 2009 (Moen, 2013; Moen et al., 2012, 2013, 2014a, 2014b; Mmbaga et al., 2012, 2014, 2017, 2018, 2020; Magesa & Leshabari, 2017; Ishungisa et al., 2020a, 2020b; National AIDS Control Programme, 2018).

The actors we discuss in this chapter were identified through a review of data generated in the course of the abovementioned work. Given space limitations, we have restricted our exploration to ten actors: (1) hardship, (2) HIV, (3) the field of public health, (4) men's sexual practices, (5) the concept of *heshima*, (6) the concept of key populations, (7) sexual lubricants, (8) religion, (9) funding agencies, and (10) money. While it may be difficult to assess which of these actors has played the most significant role in shaping grassroots organising in Dar es Salaam over the past decade, each of them has certainly made a significant difference in one or more ways.

5.3 Ten Actors that Have Shaped Community-Based Organising Among Same-Sex Attracted Men in Dar es Salaam

5.3.1 Hardship

The first actor we will consider is the experience of material hardship. A striking feature of the grassroots organising that has emerged among same-sex attracted men in Dar es Salaam is that it was not instigated by men of money, education or prestigious positions. On the contrary, it was primarily started among men from the lower socio-economic strata of the city's population; as such, it is an activism of the poor.

In interviews with grassroots actors about what might explain this characteristic, two explanations emerged. First, men of money and position were hesitant to embrace activism because they felt it could put them at considerable disadvantage. Paul, for example, one of the activists who *did* have higher education, explained how many of his peers avoided queer organisations because they feared they could lose status, jobs and wealth. "The poor are the ones that are activists, not the rich," he asserted. "The rich ones are worried about their fathers, their employers, their customers and their money."

Second, work for community-based groups could not compete with middle-class wages or the income potential of a successful business. For less well-off men, on the other hand, grassroots organising offered attractive opportunities to earn a living. The expression *maisha magumu* is frequently encountered in the street discourse in Dar es Salaam. It literally means "a hard life" and is an expression used to refer to the experience of living with limited access to material resources. The struggles and hardship of *maisha magumu* are associated with joblessness, underpaid work, poor nutrition, and aborted schooling. In a city where *maisha magumu* is commonplace, one of the reasons why community-based organisations have grown popular among poor men is the potential they represent for at least some income.

Jepther, for example, had been out of work for years when he was hired as a peer educator for one of the grassroots organisations in Dar es Salaam. He had been trying to make ends meet with a combination of the money he could generate from *kukopesha vipodozi* (selling make-up on credit), contributions from friends, and through relations with men, but it had nonetheless always been a struggle to pay the rent on time for the single room he stayed in. When he secured a position as a peer educator with one of the grassroots groups in Dar es Salaam, he was paid around 100,000 shillings (equivalent to USD43) per month. While far from enough to sustain a comfortable city life, the position came with opportunities for additional income, not least the allowances that were often paid during participation in courses and workshops arranged by NGOs and governmental agencies. Although he did not make a fortune, Jephter's newfound work provided him with a radically more predictable financial situation than he had had in the past.

Personal experience with hardship and poverty has clearly contributed to shape the activism among sexuality diverse men in Dar es Salaam. The interpersonal closeness between grassroots actors and the community members their work was aiming to support was striking. Jephter's actions as a peer educator serve to illustrate this. On a hot and humid day in 2014, the first author, as part of his fieldwork, joined Jephter while he was doing outreach in his catchment area. He was making home calls in an area of *uswahilini*, a term used to refer to neighbourhoods characterized by precarious socio-economic conditions. Most of the houses were dilapidated, and residents were struggling to make ends meet, much like Jephter himself before becoming a peer educator. His task now was to share knowledge about HIV with same-sex attracted men in this neighbourhood, to distribute condoms and lubricants to them, and to link them to friendly healthcare providers. Jepther asked the first author if they could visit one more person before lunch:

> (Summary of fieldnotes:) Jephter said: "Isaac called me yesterday and asked whether I had lubricants to share. He is a sex worker, really; he badly needs that lube." When we reached his house, Isaac was not in, but one of his neighbours told us that we were expected. She asked us to go inside and wait for him in the room he rented. We sat down on Isaac's bed in the small space. Apart from that bed, the room only contained a table, a closet, and a shelf on which there was a soap bar, a tube of skin lightening cream and a container with make-up powder. On the table lay a photo album, which Jephter opened, saying he wanted to show me Isaac's husband. He flipped through the pages and stopped at a photo of a tall, handsome man. I felt uneasy being shown this and other private photos, but Jephter clearly took for granted that it was okay to share them with me. Just then, Isaac entered the room, and he did not at all seem to mind. He smiled and greeted Jephter "*mambo vipi, shosti yangu*". The first part of this expression was the friendly, informal greeting that you may offer a close friend in street-language Swahili, whereas the *shosti yangu* he added at the end was an affectionate term meaning "my good friend." Significantly, however, it connotes femininity, and is used among women—and *magei.* Jephter pulled out 30 condoms and 10 sachets of sexual lubricant from his backpack. He handed them to Isaac, saying "I am sorry I don't have more than these ten to give you. I tried to get you some extra, but there is a shortage of lube in the office, so they limit us to ten per person." He went on to explain how it was possible to ration the lube. Since the sachets were big, one pack could suffice for two or three intercourses if the gel was applied sparingly. "But you have to fold the sachet tight in between each usage, otherwise that stuff dries up," he added, and then: "but I am telling you, do not save on the lube if the cock is big, or else you will have bruises." Isaac laughed, turned around and put the goods into his closet. A conversation about safer sex followed. Jephter and Isaac agreed that condom-protected sex was important, that *mabwana* [men; referring to the penetrating partner in gender-structured same-sex sex] did not always want to use them, but that lube was popular and made condoms more agreeable. Isaac then posed a question I had heard on many occasions before: whether lube yielded protection on its own, in the absence of condoms?

Among the things that best characterized Jephter's work was his intimate knowledge of the poor neighbourhood where he worked. He lived in a similar neighbourhood himself and had embodied knowledge of the living conditions that prevailed. Another prominent characteristic was how well he had come to know his clients; illustratively to the extent that he felt confident showing Isaac's private photo album to the first author. Perhaps more striking than anything else, however, was the sense of equivalence that characterised his interaction with his clients. Jephter clearly spoke to Isaac as his equal. The tone was light-hearted, his attitude respectful and unjudgmental, and his language straightforward and unashamed.

Freire's (1996) asserted that education needs to be based in genuine dialogue if it is to change the world in ways that benefit the oppressed. According to Freire, to engage in such dialogue presupposes equality amongst dialogical partners, and that these partners have mutual respect and even a degree of love for each other. Moreover, learners need to cultivate their own growth through situations from their daily lives that provide useful learning experiences. This would seem to be exactly the kind of education Jephter was engaging in.

The opportunities for learning and growth provided by Jephter and other peer educators in Dar es Salaam were widely appreciated among same-sex attracted men. During interviews, many talked about the ways in which they had been assisted by grassroots actors. However, grassroots activists were also criticised in the wider community of same-sex attracted men. Indeed, there was a prominent discourse that critiqued activists for being more motivated by their own well-being than by that of their clients. Michael, for example, suggested that grassroots actors were almost entirely focused on personal gain.

> Kåre, those activists receive big salaries and get to travel abroad and stay in beautiful hotels. But what are they doing to help people here? Nothing. I have not seen them do anything. Did any of them help Hamisi when he was in hospital, dying of AIDS? They did not even go to see him.

Alex's HIV infection had been detected late, and he had developed Kaposi's sarcoma only months after starting antiretroviral treatment. Although cancer medication was supposed to be free of charge in public hospitals, the medicine Alex needed was out of stock, and he had been told to buy the cytostatic himself. It cost much more than he could raise on his own. He sold his television and moved further out of town to save on his room rent, but he was entirely dependent on others if he were to access the long-term treatment that was needed. He failed in his attempts to obtain the needed funds. When he requested assistance from some of the grassroots groups, none of them had available money to pay for his treatment. He died before he had reached the age of 30.

In sum, grassroots organising among same-sex attracted men in Dar es Salaam has been fundamentally shaped by the experiences and effects of *maisha magumu* over the past decade. Many men lived precarious lives and a lack of money restricted the scope and reach of grassroots groups in a multitude of ways. At the same time, many grassroots actors had personal experience with hardship, which contributed to shape their activism in remarkable ways. Much of their work was informed by and sympathetic with precarious life conditions, and many peer educators engaged in teaching and counselling that was genuinely dialogical in style. While much of this work was widely appreciated in the queer community, there was also a discourse that critiqued grassroots activists. Grassroots work represented a valuable source of income for them, and some suggested that activists might be more motivated by opportunities for personal gain than by the collective good of the community.

5.3.2 The Human Immunodeficiency Virus

The second actor we will consider is HIV itself. The prevalence of the virus among same-sex attracted men in Dar es Salaam was unknown when grassroots organising started. Despite the lack of epidemiological data, there was obviously a significant ongoing HIV epidemic. During ethnographic fieldwork in 2008 and 2009, same-sex attracted men themselves shared knowledge of this epidemic via the narration of accumulated social and corporeal experiences (Moen, 2013). Some men had known for a long time that they were living with HIV, others tested positive while fieldwork was ongoing, many had friends who were HIV positive, and very few had not lost *gei* friends to AIDS. In some parts of Dar es Salaam, there had been so many deaths among same-sex attracted men that surviving peers could point out voids in the landscape to illustrate the impact of the ongoing epidemic. In 2009, the first author was joining a study participant on a walk through the neighbourhood in which he lived. The study participant paused at a street corner and pointed to four houses that were visible from where they were standing. A *shoga*[1] had lived in each of them, and all of them were now dead.

Furthermore, there were unmistakable indications of a significant HIV epidemic among same-sex practicing men in the literature. In 1982, the first case of HIV in a citizen of the Soviet Union was diagnosed in a homosexual man who had become HIV positive in Tanzania (Pokrovskiĭ et al., 1992). In the 1990s, an autopsy study of HIV-positive persons in Dar es Salaam reported that one-fifth of examined subjects had been homosexually exposed to HIV (Ng'walali et al., 2005). And in 2005, the first queer-identified community-based group that was established in Tanzania expressed concern about HIV and the lack of HIV prevention efforts among men who have sex with men in the country (International Capital Corporation Limited & The Gays and Lesbians of Zimbabwe, 2004). By 2008, however, there was still no programmes that addressed HIV among same-sex practising men, nor did local and international agencies have plans for such work.

When the first epidemiological data were gathered, the significant HIV epidemic among men who have sex with men in Dar es Salaam was confirmed. A study carried out in 2012 reported an HIV prevalence of 30.2% among such men (Ross et al., 2014), while a larger study in 2014 found the HIV prevalence among men who have sex with men in Dar es Salaam to be 22.3% (Mmbaga et al., 2018). At this particular point in time, the overall HIV prevalence in Tanzania was on the decline. It had fallen from 7.0% in 2004 to 5.1% in 2012 (Tanzania Commission for AIDS, 2013). The likelihood that a same-sex practising man was HIV positive, therefore, was four to six times higher than among adults in general.

As these statistics became available, the community-based groups shared them with their constituencies. While activists had no doubt that they were facing a

[1]*Shoga* is a term referring to a category of same-sex practising men; typically expected to have womanly qualities and take a penetrated corporeal position in a same-sex sexual encounter. In mainstream discourse, this term is often used interchangeably with *gei*.

considerable HIV epidemic even before it was documented by epidemiologists, the proportions reported seemed entirely overwhelming. At a meeting called by one of the grassroots groups in 2013, many activists expressed a sense of alarm. One of those present exclaimed, "If we do not do much more, we will all die."

While antiretroviral treatment was available in Dar es Salaam by this point in time, HIV infection was still associated with serious consequences, including death. The lay knowledge that circulated among grassroots actors was that many deaths from HIV were linked to the conditions of *maisha magumu*. Poor men had insufficient diets, and this was associated with mortality both directly and indirectly, as it could be highly unpleasant to take antiretroviral drugs on an empty stomach.

In sum, a dramatic HIV epidemic has informed and animated grassroots organising among same-sex attracted men in Dar es Salaam over the past decade. HIV prevention programming targeting this population was severely delayed, and HIV prevalence rates rose to four to six times higher than in the overall adult population in the first half of the 2010s. Even in the presence of ART, burials of men who had HIV continued to be a common occurrence, linked to the many ill effects of *maisha magumu*.

5.3.3 The Field of Public Health

The third actor we want to consider is the field of public health, a discipline that understands itself as one that "promotes and protects the health of people and the communities where they live, learn, work and play" (American Public Health Association, 2019). Notwithstanding this self-understanding, public health was a largely absent actor in HIV prevention with and among same-sex attracted men on much of the African continent for two decades after the epidemic emerged. Let us stress that this absence did not only pertain to African practitioners of public health but was a feature of the global public health community's response to HIV in Africa. For years, key global actors seemed to take for granted that male-to-male sexual relations had next to nothing to do with HIV in Africa. An early authoritative text like *AIDS in the World* (Mann et al., 1992), for example, discussed same-sex sex at length in its chapters on Europe and the U.S.A., but limited itself to noting that "very little" was known about same-sex practices in the context of the African HIV epidemic. More knowledge did not seem to be urgently needed, moreover: the book did not call for any knowledge production on this front. Not until 2005, more than 20 years into the pandemic, was the first HIV seroprevalence study among African men who have sex with other men carried out (in Senegal; Wade et al., 2005). Just as in Dar es Salaam a few years later, this study found considerably higher HIV prevalence among same-sex attracted men than among other adults.

While the public health response was severely delayed in Dar es Salaam, the field of public health did eventually come to play a role in the emergence of community-based organising among same-sex attracted men. The initial contribution was rather indirect, but significant nonetheless. Two grassroots organisations were established in 2010 by men who had worked as research assistants for various HIV-related research projects focusing on men who have sex with other men. Many of the men came from backgrounds where *maisha magumu* prevailed, including James, a founding member of one of these groups. When the project he had been employed by came to an end, he and a few colleagues vowed to start a community-based organisation with the aim of "fighting AIDS" among same-sex attracted men. In interviews, some of these men pointed to the knowledge they had gained as public health research assistants as an important reason for starting the new organisations. They had also been exposed to persons and organisations in HIV programming that proved important as their community-based work got under way.

As public health research focusing on HIV among same-sex attracted men got under way in Dar es Salaam, it was applauded by many community members. As part of the "Dar es Salaam MSM study" in 2014, we conducted follow-on qualitative research to explore study participants' perceptions of the study. A striking finding was that many men thought of the research as a sign of inclusion and acceptance of queer subjects. Two of the interviewees put it this way:

> What the university is doing is something great when they receive people of our kind, which is something other institutions have not managed to do.

> The gays are hearing about this study, and what they get from it is that it is possible to go to the hospital and you will not be discriminated. I believe this will give courage to those who are worried to see a doctor.

Despite positive feedback of this kind, the field of public health has also been sternly critiqued by queer activists in Dar es Salaam; a criticism we will return to shortly. For now, we note that considered as an actor in community-based organising among same-sex attracted men in Dar es Salaam, the field of public health was disturbingly absent for a long time. Eventually, however, it contributed to facilitate a new era of grassroots organising. Significant new grassroots groups were established by men who had worked as assistants in public health research into HIV among same-sex attracted men, and the public health research itself that focused on HIV among same-sex attracted men was perceived to provide symbolic and moral support.

5.3.4 Sexual Practices and Their HIV-Related Risks

As a fourth actor that contributed to shape community-based organising in the past decade, let us briefly consider the sexual practices that same-sex attracted men in Dar es Salaam engaged in, and the HIV-related risks that were inherent in them. The Dar es Salaam MSM study (Mmbaga et al., 2014, 2018) found that sexual debut among same-sex practising men in the city occurred at a young age (one quarter of men had had their initial sexual experience before the age of 15), that bisexual practices were more common than strictly same-sex practices (84% of men had ever had a female partner), and that sexual position taking was typically fixed (only 7% of respondents reported engaging in both insertive and receptive anal sex). Just over a quarter had ever engaged in group sex, and 7% had engaged in such sex over the past 3 months.

While many of these practices entailed potential risk for HIV acquisition and transmission, protected sex was comparatively uncommon. A condom was used in less than half of all sexual encounters, but more often in male-to-male sex (45% had used a condom during their last male to male sexual encounter) than in sexual encounters with women (27% of men who had sex with both men and women had used a condom in their last sexual encounter with a woman). Significantly, moreover, only one third of respondents had ever used a water-based lubricant, and when asked about access to lube, a large majority said that it was difficult to get hold of.

Informed by embodied and theoretical knowledge about sexual practices and their risks, many of the grassroots group in Dar es Salaam in the middle of the 2010s focused on the promotion of safer sex. Making sexual lubricants available was one priority area of this work. As we will discuss shortly, this was associated with considerable controversy.

5.3.5 *Heshima*

The fifth actor we will consider is the concept of *heshima*. This concept is central to Tanzanian discourse on appropriate conduct and means "to have dignity, honour, and respect, as well as knowing how to properly extend courtesy and esteem to others" (McMahon, 2006). *Heshima* has played a significant role in many aspects of community-based organising among same-sex attracted men in Dar es Salaam. The way Jephter carried out his tasks as a peer educator, for example, was informed and shaped by codes for respectful dialogue, as was the way he acted in relation to the leader of the organisation for which he worked, a topic we will return to. However, the issue of *heshima* took on a particularly significant role in considerations about how community-based groups should interact with the wider public and the authorities about issues pertaining to same-sex sexualities.

The high HIV prevalence rates among same-sex attracted men in Dar es Salaam alarmed queer community groups, and the case for a more dedicated HIV response seemed urgent. Some activists argued powerfully for considerably more involvement from national and local leaders. As Ambokile, one of the grassroots actors, put it:

> ... how can this country get to zero unless more is done to prevent HIV among MSM? Everyone is talking about zero, but among gays HIV is a hundred more than it is zero. ... Until the leaders do something, we are doomed. So that's why we need to apply for money to do sensitization of politicians.

Ambokile's idea was to engage with the polity to make the point that better HIV prevention among same-sex attracted men was urgently needed, and to do this within a framework that entailed an explicit human rights agenda along with the focus on HIV.

While many grassroots actors supported activism of this type, others did not. Those who were sceptical argued that rights-based activism might stir up controversy. Jackson, for example, was adamant that a politicisation of gay issues and rights was not a good idea at all,

> Most of the leaders have no problem with gays. They just want to keep us out of politics, and they are right. It has never been a problem being gay in Tanzania, but I am telling you, if you bring us into politics, there will be big problems. ... Just look at Uganda.

In Uganda, one of Tanzania's neighbouring countries, the issue of homosexuality had been a hotly debated political issue since 2009 (e.g., Tamale, 2009; Strand, 2011; Semugoma et al., 2012). The situation in Tanzania was radically different at the time. Although there was stigma and discrimination against same-sex attracted men, there was also palpable acceptance of same-sex attraction and gender variation in the wider community. Furthermore, few if any politicians had paid attention to the issue of homosexuality over the years, either positively or negatively, at least not in public. Some grassroots actors reasoned that the latter fact reflected a widely shared norm proscribing open conversation about sex and sexuality in formal contexts.

> It is not that they do not know! They know, of course, and some of them are gays themselves. But to discuss sex openly in politics would be a disaster. It does not belong there. (Baraka)

Baraka's point was that although there was tacit acceptance of same-sex relations in strata of the population as well as in strata of the polity, such relations did not belong in public discourse. Homosexuality was not an issue so long as it did not erupt into discourses where it did not belong. As Shukuru explained:

> You cannot do that in Tanzania. It will not be understood. I have never talked to my parents about being gay. They know that, of course: I have never had a girlfriend and all my gay friends know my mother; come on. But I would have no *heshima* if I started talking about sex with my parents. It has nothing to do with being gay; even my brothers and sisters should not talk about sex with our parents. [...] And now you want to tell me that we should discuss sex with the leaders of the nation? It is not possible. Do not force the topic, it cannot go well.

To introduce homosexuality into explicit public discussion, in Shukuru's view, entailed a predictable outcome. He reasoned that nothing good could come out of it, and he feared that the implicit acceptance of same-sex relations would be at risk. Although Shukuru's views were criticised as conservative among some grassroots actors, many groups nonetheless took a rather careful approach to activism, trying to avoid media attention, and making sure their focus was on health and not on rights.

The topic of same-sex sexualities has nonetheless gained considerable political attention in recent years, culminating with massive national and international media coverage of same-sex issues in Tanzanian politics in 2017 and 2018. Among other things, a previous government minister warned that campaigners for gay rights should face punitive measures (Ng'wanakilala, 2017), and the regional commissioner of Dar es Salaam called on members of the public to report homosexuals to the authorities (Gloppen & Rakner, 2019). There was considerable concern among queer activists as these situations unfolded, and some left Dar es Salaam due to safety concerns. A few days after the regional commissioner's statements, however, the government made clear that they did not reflect any official position, and that Tanzania would "continue to respect all international human rights conventions which it subscribes to" (AFP, 2018). Notwithstanding this, some community-based groups that have been involved in HIV related grassroots work were deregistered by the Non-Governmental Organisations Coordination Board in 2019, reportedly for "promoting unethical acts which violates Tanzanian ethics, laws and culture" (The Citizen, 2019).

In sum, *heshima* has been a significant actor in queer grassroots organising in Dar es Salaam. As a norm, it compels citizens to abstain from bringing sexual topics into respectful discourse. While open, free and explicit talk about sex and sexualities is commonplace in a wide range of informal settings, this prescription acted to make many grassroots actors aware that communicating about same-sex attracted men and their circumstances in public debate required a high level of care. There has been ongoing controversy among grassroots activists about how best to deal with these issues. Some warned vehemently against grassroots action that could elicit responses like the ones that have been reported in recent years, whereas others were of the opinion that challenging such responses was needed to build a stronger response to the HIV epidemic among men who have sex with men.

5.3.6 The Concept of Key Populations

Notwithstanding the relative paucity of political debate about same-sex practices until recent years, Tanzanian official policy has addressed the situation for men who have sex with men since 2003. The first National Multisectoral Framework on HIV/AIDS (The Prime Minister's Office, 2003) called for research into HIV-related vulnerabilities among men who have sex with other men, and later documents encouraged HIV programming for this segment of the population. These policies have increasingly been articulated in the language of "key populations," a concept promoted globally by entities such as the WHO, UNAIDS and PEPFAR. The first Tanzanian "National Guideline for a Comprehensive Package of HIV Interventions for Key Populations" was issued in 2014 (National AIDS Control Programme, 2014) and revised in 2016. The sixth actor we will consider is the core concept in these policy documents; namely, that of key populations.

In the WHO definition (2014), key populations are "groups who, due to specific higher-risk behaviours, are at increased risk of HIV irrespective of the epidemic type or local context" (p. xiv) who "often have legal and social issues related to their behaviours that increase their vulnerability to HIV" (ibid.). The term is taken to include men who have sex with men, people who inject drugs, persons who sell sex and transgender people. As this term gained ground in Dar es Salaam over the past decade, it became so widely adopted that some same-sex attracted men started to refer to themselves, individually and collectively, as "key populations". Many also used the abbreviation KP for this purpose, and expressions such as "we KPs" and "I am a KP" became commonplace.

Many grassroots actors found the KP term helpful. Among other things, it was an expression that could make them both visible and concealed. Because it was rather vague and ambiguous, it was not associated with much controversy, and because it did not make explicit reference to sexual identity, it was a way of talking about the circumstances of same-sex attracted men in formal discourse that did not so easily conflict with the principle of *heshima*.

Another aspect of the concept that was celebrated among some grassroots actors was the sense of solidarity that came along with it. Said Innocent, one of the grassroots activists:

> A good thing [about KP] is that all of those that were left by the roadside are now put together. When you talk about KP, you cannot help one group and leave the others aside.

While there was broad adoption of the concept of key populations among queer grassroots actors, there were also critical views. Among them, the concept was thought to encourage a conflation of highly different populations and could lead to the idea that identical approaches to HIV programming were relevant for all of them. For example, some public health professionals were said to conflate same-sex attracted men and drug users with respect to the strategies that could and should be used to promote HIV prevention among them. Explained Willam:

> Many of them [public health programmers] keep asking us "how many have you managed to stop from that behaviour," meaning whether we have stopped men from having sex with men.

While the abandonment of drug use was a relatively uncontroversial aim in HIV programming with people who use drugs, queer grassroots actors found it upsetting that some public health professionals were of the view that the relinquishment of same-sex sexual practices should be a goal for HIV programming among same-sex attracted men. Combining these two diverse groups into a single KP category enabled conservative public health actors to advocate against same-sex relations with the rationale of preventing HIV.

The concept of key populations therefore both enabled and complicated queer grassroots organising in Dar es Salaam. On the one hand, the concept provided policymakers, public health practitioners and grassroots actors with a language that was acceptable in wide circles, and thereby allowed discourse that might otherwise have been considered controversial. On the other hand, since the concept of key populations at times was used to conflate diverse populations, it was also perceived to promote ideas about the erasure of same-sex sexual practices.

5.3.7 *Sexual Lube*

As we have already alluded to, sexual lubricants were an actor that intervened considerably with grassroots organising to prevent HIV among same-sex attracted men in Dar es Salaam. As mentioned, only a fraction of them had personal experience with water and silicone-based lubricants in the mid-2010s. As part of grassroots efforts to promote safer sex, organizations emphasized advocacy for consistent condom use together with appropriate lubrication, in line with long-standing public health recommendations. HIV prevention programming guidelines for men who have sex with men have promoted the use of sexual lubricants for decades. The *Consolidated guidelines on HIV prevention, diagnosis, treatment and care for key populations* (WHO, 2014), for example, emphasises that condoms should not be promoted alone, but in tandem with sexual lubricants because condoms easily break or slip off during anal sex in the absence of appropriate lubrication.

Given such recommendations, lube might seem likely to be an uncontroversial actor in HIV programming. However, things do not always perform in predictable ways. In the lingo of Latour (2007), lube did not act as an "intermediary," but rather as a "mediator;" an entity that can modify, translate and sometimes distort meaning. Indeed, tiny packets of slippery stuff became a controversial sign in ongoing efforts to prevent HIV among same-sex practising men in Tanzania. According to grassroots actors in 2014, the national entity regulating the quality and safety of medical products did not permit the import of sexual lubricants, requiring that they first be tested for safety. Some activists contacted regulatory representatives to inquire and reported that they were told that lubricants were unacceptable because they promoted homosexuality. Subsequently, the accuracy of this claim was discussed among grassroots actors. Some argued that persons who desire to engage in same-sex sex would do so whether they have access to water-based lube or not, whereas others argued that the regulators might perhaps have a point. Since anal sex in the absence of lubrication can be painful for the penetrated partner, lubricants might perhaps be considered capable of facilitating the occurrence of this form of sex.

Notwithstanding this, grassroots actors felt compelled to prevent HIV transmission by making lube available. Therefore, a group of activists travelled to neighbouring Kenya to purchase as much lube as they could afford. They brought it back as travel luggage on a bus. At the border, customs officers had to be "tipped" in order to get the consignment across, but finally the boxes of lube arrived at the office, where it was rationed and peer educators like Jephter were authorized to provide 10 sachets a time.

A few weeks later, the issue of lube and *gei* organising suddenly made it to the newspapers. One of the tabloids published an interview with an anonymous man who claimed he had been lured into the offices of one of the grassroots organisations in Dar es Salaam. He reportedly described it as a place where people had sex with each other and explained that activists had tried to entice him into sexual activity. Further critical media reporting followed, focusing, among other things, on the Facebook page of the organisation, where there were photos of the lube that the organisation was distributing, allegedly in order to promote anal sex. A few days later, authority representatives made an unannounced visit to the organisation's office and asked for the registration documents while they evaluated the situation. Eventually, they found a discrepancy between the group's registered objectives and the actual activities carried out. While the organisation was registered as an HIV prevention group, its activity profile was found to promote homosexuality, and it was eventually deregistered.

As an actor, lube was very versatile in Dar es Salaam. A gel-like substance packaged in tiny sachets was strong enough to prevent HIV, but also to promote homosexuality. At any rate, it encouraged grassroots activists to break the law in the name of HIV prevention and led to the deregistration of community-based groups that worked to prevent HIV among same-sex attracted men.

5.3.8 Religion

Another actor that interfered with grassroots organising among same-sex attracted men in Dar es Salaam was religion. As in many places across the world, same-sex relations got entangled in debates about sin and immorality in mainstream Christian and Muslim discourse, and same-sex attracted men explained how some churches offered gay men opportunities to 'leave their habits'.

Religious perspectives on same-sex relations from time to time also made it to the media, for example through media coverage of *anti* Asu,[2] a famous *shoga* who had been "born again" and—coinciding with this—healed from homosexuality (Kajuna, 2013). In the past, anti Asu had been a well-known figure on Dar es Salaam's club scene, and they had often made it to the gossip columns of the tabloids. The media attention had mostly focused on their elegant female attire. The contrast was dramatic when the new images of a stout man clad in a suit and tie appeared in the newspapers. The person previously known as anti Asu appeared on talk shows on the radio as well, on one occasion giving out their phone number so that *magei* might get in touch and be helped in the same way they had been. Grassroots actors discussed and criticised these developments, and plentiful stories circulated about what had happened. Among them was a rumour that anti Asu had received considerable incentives, including cash and a car, from the church in exchange for their transformation.

While both Christian and Muslim leaders were associated with critique of same-sex practices, it is important to point out that there were also signs of acceptance and support of same-sex attracted men and their grassroots organising from within religious circles. Significantly, the most popular health provider among same-sex attracted men in Dar es Salaam was a clinic owned and operated by a church. It provided dedicated services to men who have sex with men and received wide-ranging praise in the queer community.

[2]*Anti* is a Swahilification of the English "auntie".

5.3.9 Funders

The ninth actor we will consider is funding agencies and mechanisms for grassroots work. As mentioned, many of the grassroots groups in Dar es Salaam were initiated by men without plentiful material resources. When they started their work, they typically had little or no money whatsoever. There was no budget, no allowances, and no offices to work from. Initially, the activists from one of the groups met in a bar that was rather quiet during daytime. They purchased their first used laptop with money or that had been donated by themselves and some of their cash-strapped peers. The organisation was able to hire an office when they won a start-up grant from an NGO in another African country that operated a funding scheme for queer grassroots organisations. A grand total of USD3500 was transferred to the group's newly established bank account. While the amount was modest, it made a huge difference by allowing the group to rent an office, purchase a second computer and illegally import a few boxes of sexual lubricants.

Nevertheless, more resources were needed, and grant proposal writing soon became a main activity in the office. One morning in 2014, ten or so people were crammed together in one room. They were sitting in two circles, each surrounding a laptop computer. On both, a funding proposal was under preparation. The room was buzzing with voices; intense discussions were ongoing in Swahili, a language that all of those present excelled in. The writing, however, was carried out in English, a language only a few mastered. In Tanzania, English is the medium of instruction in secondary schools and universities, whereas Swahili is used in primary schools. The activists had diverse backgrounds, but as we have mentioned, only a few had higher education. Their activism was anchored in a wide variety of lived experiences as same-sex attracted men. The experiences and insights these men had accumulated could be well articulated, celebrated and problematized in Swahili, and in the range of other languages the activists spoke (Tanzania has 164 or so different idioms). However, few were the funding organisations that could speak—or who would allow correspondence in—any of these. On the contrary, proposals had to be written in the colonial language that many years earlier had been used to compose the law that still forbade "carnal knowledge against the order of nature" in Tanzania (United Republic of Tanzania, 1998) and many other former countries of the British empire (Human Rights Watch, 2008; Ottosson, 2010).

To write proposals was therefore a time-consuming process, and in addition, one that included a considerable amount of second-guessing what the donor would like to hear. Among the consequences of the foreign language requirement, moreover, was that most ideas had to be extensively discussed before they could be put on paper. Whereas an acronym like LGBTIQ may flow easily, and without much reflection from the keyboard of activists in English-speaking countries in the West, the conundrum of this letter combination was fully revealed among activists who tried to make sense of it within the framework of a different language and a different set of sexual cultures. After several hours of work on a proposal that was to be submitted to a foreign funding agency, the activists first concluded that they wanted to describe their organisation as a "GBT group;" G for gay, B for bisexual, and T for transsexual. This decision was thereafter amended since that three-letter combination excluded SW for sex workers, of which there were perceived to be many among GBT in Dar es Salaam. In the end, therefore, the agreement was to add SW to the row of letters so that the proposal came to address GBTSW people.

Apart from the language requirement, most funding organisations demanded that templates be used when preparing funding proposals. As part of the template for the GBTSW application, a "problem tree" needed to be developed to provide an overview of the problems the organisation faced and how these were interlinked. Smaller twigs were to represent specific problems, which were to sprout from larger stems representing underlying causes and difficulties. The problem tree encouraged the proposal writers to strive to identify and articulate as many problems as possible. In the course of this process, competencies, insights and strengths silently retreated into the background, and their work came to be re-represented in terms of deficiencies and absences. Among the problems the grassroots actors listed were a lack of organisational skills, a lack of insight into LGBTI issues, a lack of knowledge about HIV, a lack of familiarity with HIV prevention, too little experience, a lack of education, deficient safety and security, weak stakeholder support, a shortage of computers, insufficient management skills, weak communication abilities, a deficiency of language competencies, and a scarcity of communication materials. While many of the issues that were described as deficiencies were not unimportant challenges, the problem tree came to make the organisation look awfully resource-deficient. Asked about this by the first author, the activists agreed it made them look bad, but their impression was that donor organisations were interested in weak organisations. Unless you articulated problems that made you seem worthy of assistance, there would be no way you would be successful in your funding request.

Considered as an actor, funding agencies clearly contributed to make grassroots action possible in Dar es Salaam. With relatively modest sums of money, funders enabled grassroots organisations to get established, hire staff, purchase equipment and carry out their activities. At the same time, funders often seemed ill-prepared to engage with grassroots activism of the type that occurred in Dar es Salaam. By setting foreign language requirements and demanding the use of templates that did not take into consideration the cultural context in which the funding was supposed to be of assistance, funders also created a considerable extra workload for grassroots actors and caused insecurity and confusion. Many funders were perceived to view grassroots actors in terms of their weaknesses rather in terms of their strengths and resources.

5.3.10 Money

The tenth and final actor we will consider is the money that grassroots groups were able to attract through funding mechanisms described in the previous section, and the market-like conditions and challenges that such money brought into grassroots organising. While funding was needed to allow community action to occur, the "invisible hand" of the market also led to competition, conflict and the advent of a class-divided community in miniature.

Accessing funding was often competitive. At times, the competition was fought through proposal writing, as discussed in the previous section, but making oneself stand out to donors and their representatives was often important as well. When a foreign NGO was going to initiate HIV programming in key populations in Dar es Salaam a few years ago, for example, it set in motion a process aiming to identify and team up with a suitable "MSM-led" community-based group. The process was to culminate with the selection of a single partner, and this put pressure on grassroots groups in Dar es Salaam to present themselves in the best possible light. In addition, however, groups also got entangled in struggles to discredit each other. Stories about the shortcomings and weaknesses of competing groups multiplied and included claims about mismanagement of funds and that competing organisations were "fake" in the sense that their activists claimed to be gay when they actually were not. Because of processes like this, the climate between grassroots groups in Dar es Salaam at times became severely strained.

As entrepreneurs, as it were, in a marketplace of queer programming, community-based groups were also subject to the unpredictability of market forces. Funding was typically made available for short-term projects, and the future of each grassroots group was continuously in danger as a result. The market insecurity was at times acute. In 2014, for example, one of the funders suddenly discontinued its payments to the organisations it supported. The explanation offered was that money from an external donor was delayed. It was asserted that funding would resume later, and the organisations were requested to continue their work in the interim. Some of them did not have a financial reserve that could pay salaries in lieu of the funder and had to pass on the consequences of the delay to its employees. Although there was no payment forthcoming for 6 months, the activists did not stop their activities. In what can only be interpreted as a sign of enormous commitment to the work they were doing, grassroots actors at times even borrowed money to cover their bus fares to come to the office, and many had to deal with financial difficulties in their private lives.

In many groups, the level of income differed significantly between cadres of grassroots actors, and these differences were the source of both controversy and the emergence of what resembled class relations within the grassroots movement. Most groups had a director at the top, assisted by a wider leadership team consisting of persons with more specialised tasks (such as overseeing programming or monitoring and evaluation activities). At the bottom of the organisational hierarchy was typically a rather large number of peer educators. Many directors appeared to have a good income, but while some had a high salary, this was not always the case. Indeed, some directors did not take out any salary at all from their organisations but were paid what remained when an externally funded activity had been completed and all activity-related costs paid. For most peer educators, on the other hand, payment often was in the form of daily or weekly allowances rather than a salary. As mentioned earlier, while modest, the money they earned often made a significant difference in their lives. At the same time, many complained that the income difference between themselves and their directors was huge. This disparity was also observable in social life, along with what could be interpreted as an emerging social class formation among grassroots activists. Persons in the upper tier of this class system gathered in posh bars and clubs, whereas "working class" activists went to cheaper places or did not go out much at all. If they did come to the high-class venues, they often could not afford drinks themselves. Many also pointed out how the upper-class activists lived in larger and nicer apartments, had fancier clothes, and engaged in discussion about luxurious goods like top-end smartphones.

In comparison with the standards of the upper middle class in Dar es Salaam, or those of foreign NGO representatives, the lifestyle of the upper activist class was modest. However, the disparity between *wakubwa na wadogo* (the big and the small; about people) were nonetheless considerable, and with these differences followed suspicion about money being mismanaged, diverted and misallocated. When rumours portrayed a director's lifestyle as excessively lavish, for example, they were regularly accompanied by incisive questions: Where had the money come from? How much? Who else had been involved? The most interesting aspect of these stories is perhaps not whether they were always true or not, but the way in which they revealed a sense of social disparity among the human actors engaging in grassroots organising in Dar es Salaam. This, in turn, reflected market mechanisms put in place by structures, goals and powerful donors, most of which were located far away from Dar es Salaam.

In summary, the advent of community-based *gei* organisations in Dar es Salaam was associated with the emergence of a class-divided community in miniature. At the top of each organisation was a leadership, typically consisting of persons with considerably better pay than the peer educators, who constituted the working class of grassroots activism.

5.4 Discussion

While working on this chapter, the first author encountered a representative of an international non-governmental organisation (INGO) which provides support to queer community-based organising across the world. Upon learning the subject of this chapter, he did not hesitate to offer the opinion that queer grassroots organising in Dar es Salaam was "weak". He had only been to Dar es Salaam once (for a 2-day stay at one of the conference beach hotels) but referred to colleagues and impressions circulating in the queer-oriented INGO world as the background for this evaluation. Among the critical remarks he shared was that grassroots organisations in Dar es Salaam had been unable to develop a strong rights agenda, that they had weak leaders, that they were no good at advocacy, that they were infamous for financial mismanagement, that they had not been able to work together to any large extent, and that they were lacking in competence and capacity. On the background of impressions like this, his organisation was planning to seek funding that would allow them to run capacity building workshops in Dar es Salaam.

Just as with the problem trees referred to earlier, this list of deficiencies made the grassroots actors in Dar es Salaam look awfully inadequate. However, while imperfect, inadequacy is hardly the most striking characteristic of grassroots actors in Dar es Salaam. Indeed, it is much more remarkable how they have been able to initiate and sustain their efforts over the past decade. If an actor is what is made to act by many others, it would seem possible, perhaps even likely, that the grassroots movement in Tanzania's largest city had come to wrap up their act altogether over the past decade. Many agents have seemed inclined to make them do exactly that, including the field of public health that ignored same-sex attracted men for such a long time, the overwhelming HIV epidemic that would appear to be closely related to this ignoring, the concept of key populations that promoted the idea that sexual lives should perhaps be erased in efforts to control HIV, the homosexuality-promoting agency of lube, the funding agencies that were more focused on the sharing of their own templates than on learning from actors on the ground, and the community disruption that followed from the emergence of a marketplace of sorts for grassroots organising. However, rather than succumbing to factors such as these, grassroots actors in Dar es Salaam have been able to adapt and multiply their community-based work. By drawing on the values inherent in *heshima*, they have found allies in unexpected places (e.g., in the church), practiced reasoned subversion (e.g. by establishing alternative lube supply lines), and created widespread community awareness and action through dialogical education.

Significantly, at the start of the 2020s, the tide of the HIV epidemic among same-sex attracted men in Dar es Salaam seems to have turned. A recent study suggests that there has been a considerable reduction in the HIV prevalence among same-sex attracted men in Dar es Salaam over the past few years. While almost one third were HIV positive in the first half of the decade, the HIV prevalence is now below 10% (Ishungisa et al., 2020a). While there are certainly several developments that have contributed to this remarkable reduction (and many lives that have been lost), it is unimaginable that this could have been achieved without the immense dialogical effort that has been carried out by peer educators across Dar es Salaam.

Maybe the INGO that wanted to capacity build in Dar es Salaam ought to reconsider their plans? Might it not be time to focus more on learning from grassroots actors than teaching them? This is certainly what Freire (1996) would have urged them to do. His insight was that all education needs to be based in genuine dialogue if it is to change the world in ways that benefit the oppressed. To engage in such dialogue presupposes equality amongst partners, and that partners have mutual love and respect for each other. Moreover, learners need to cultivate their own growth through situations from their daily lives that provide useful learning experiences, which is just what grassroots organisations have been able to do to contribute to bringing down the prevalence among same-sex attracted men.

References

Agence France-Presse. (2018). *Tanzania government denounces Makonda's anti-gay clampdown.* Retrieved July 6, 2019, from https://www.theeastafrican.co.ke/news/ea/Tanzania-government-denounces-Makonda-anti-gay-clampdown/4552908-4837714-m0w84v/index.html

American Public Health Association. (2019). *What is public health?* Retrieved July 6, 2019, from https://www.apha.org/what-is-public-health

Collins, C. J., Greenall, M. N., Mallouris, C., & Smith, S. L. (2016). Time for full inclusion of community actions in the response to AIDS. *Journal of the International AIDS Society, 19*(1), 20712.

Freire, P. (1996). *Pedagogy of the oppressed (revised).* Continuum.

Gloppen, S. R., & Rakner, L. (2019). *The perfect enemy: From migrants to sexual minorities.* Chr. Michelsen Institute. Retrieved July 6, 2019, from https://www.cmi.no/publications/6861-the-perfect-enemy-from-migrants-to-sexual-minorities

Human Rights Watch. (2008). *This alien legacy: The origins of "sodomy" laws in British colonialism.* Human Rights Watch.

International Capital Corporation Limited, & The Gays and Lesbians of Zimbabwe. (2004, February 7–14). *All Africa symposium on HIV/AIDS and human rights.* Official report. Johannesburg.

Ishungisa, A. M., Moen, K., Leyna, G., Makyao, N., Lange, T., Meyrowitsch, D. W., et al. (2020a). HIV prevalence among men who have sex with men following the implementation of the HIV preventive guideline in Tanzania: Respondent-driven sampling survey. *BMJ Open, 10*(10), e036460.

Ishungisa, A. M., Mzinduko, M., Likindikoki, S., Mmbaga, E. J., Leshabari, M., & Moen, K. (2020b). Health services we can trust: How same-sex attracted men in Dar es Salaam, Tanzania would like their healthcare to be organized. *Culture, Health and Sexuality.* https://doi.org/10.1080/13691058.2020.1780316.

Kajuna, C. (2013). *Shoga Anti Asu Aokoka.* Retrieved July 6, 2019, from http://www.kajunason.com/2013/09/shoga-anti-asu-aokoka.html

Kameni, B. S., Nansseu, J. R., Tatah, S. A., & Bigna, J. J. (2019). Sustaining the community dispensation strategy of HIV antiretroviral through community participation. *Infectious Diseases of Poverty, 8*(1), 1–6.

Latour, B. (2007). *Reassembling the social.* Oxford University Press.

Magesa, D. J., & Leshabari, M. (2017). Perceived barriers to access available health services among men who have sex with men in Dar es Salaam, Tanzania. *Tanzania Journal of Health Research, 19.* https://doi.org/10.4314/thrb.v19i4.

Mann, J. M., Tarantola, D., & Netter, T. W. (1992). *AIDS in the world.* Harvard University Press.

McMahon, E. (2006). "A solitary tree builds not": Heshima, community, and shifting identity in post-emancipation Pemba Island. *The International Journal of African Historical Studies, 39*, 197–219.

Mmbaga, E. J., Dodo, M. J., Leyna, G. H., Moen, K., & Leshabari, M. T. (2012). Sexual practices and perceived susceptibility to HIV infection among men who have sex with men in Dar es Salaam, mainland Tanzania. *Journal of AIDS and Clinical Research, S1*, 012.

Mmbaga, E., Mpembeni, R., Leshabari, M., & Moen, K. (2014). *Prevalence of HIV, other STIs, and health-related perceptions, reflections, experiences and practices among men having sex with men in Dar es Salaam.* Muhimbili University of Health and Allied Sciences.

Mmbaga, E. J., Moen, K., Makyao, N., Mpembeni, R., & Leshabari, M. T. (2017). HIV and STI s among men who have sex with men in Dodoma municipality, Tanzania: A cross-sectional study. *Sexually Transmitted Infections, 93*, 314–319.

Mmbaga, E. J., Moen, K., Leyna, G. H., Mpembeni, R., & Leshabari, M. T. (2018). HIV prevalence and associated risk factors among men who have sex with men in Dar es Salaam, Tanzania. *Journal of the Acquired Immune Deficiency Syndrome, 77*, 243–249.

Mmbaga, E. J., Leyna, G. H., Leshabari, M. T., & Moen, K. (2020). Early anal sex experience among men who have sex with men in Dar es Salaam Tanzania: Implications for HIV prevention and care. *Archives of Sexual Behavior, 49*(6), 2045–2055.
Moen, K. (2013). *Same-sex attracted men in Tanzania 30 years into the HIV epidemic: A qualitative study*. PhD dissertation, University of Oslo.
Moen, K., Aggleton, P., Leshabari, M. T., & Middelthon, A.-L. (2012). Not at all so hard-to-reach: Same-sex attracted men in Dar es Salaam. *Culture, Health and Sexuality, 14*, 195–208.
Moen, K., Aggleton, P., Leshabari, M. T., & Middelthon, A.-L. (2013). Situating condoms in sexual lives: Experiences of same-sex-attracted men in Tanzania. *International Journal of Sexual Health, 25*, 185–197.
Moen, K., Aggleton, P., Leshabari, M. T., & Middelthon, A.-L. (2014a). Gays, guys, and mchicha mwiba: Same-sex relations and subjectivities in Dar es Salaam. *Journal of Homosexuality, 61*, 511–539.
Moen, K., Aggleton, P., Leshabari, M. T., & Middelthon, A.-L. (2014b). Same-sex practicing men in Tanzania from 1860 to 2010. *Archives of Sexual Behavior, 43*(5), 1065–1082.
National AIDS Control Programme. (2014). *National guideline for comprehensive package of HIV interventions for key populations*. National AIDS Control Programme.
National AIDS Control Programme. (2018). *Integrated bio-behavioural survey among men who have sex with men in Dar es Salaam, 2017*. Muhimbili University of Health and Allied Sciences.
National Bureau of Statistics. (2012). *2012 population and housing census*. National Bureau of Statistics.
Ng'walali, P. M., Kibayashi, K., Mbonde, M. P., Harada, S., Mwakagile, D., Kitinya, J. N., & Tsunenari, S. (2005). Neuropathology of human immunodeficiency virus infection: A forensic autopsy study in Dar es Salaam, Tanzania. *Forensic Science International, 151*, 133–138.
Ng'wanakilala, F. (2017). *Tanzania threatens crackdown on LGBT advocates*. Retrieved July 6, 2019, from https://www.reuters.com/article/tanzania-lgbt-idUSL8N1JN373
Ottosson, D. (2010). *State-sponsored homophobia. A world survey of laws prohibiting same-sex activity between consenting adults*. ILGA—The International Lesbian, Gay, Bisexual, Trans and Intersex Association. Retrieved May 1, 2012, from https://www.gaylawnet.com/ezine/crime/ilga_2010.pdf
Pokrovskiĭ, V., Iurin, O., Kravchenko, A., Potekaev, N., Gabrilovich, D., Makarova, N. I., & Potekaev, S. (1992). *[The first case of HIV infection in a citizen of the USSR] (Abstract in English)*. Retrieved October 11, 2019, from http://www.ncbi.nlm.nih.gov/pubmed/1301654
Rodriguez-García, R., Bonnel, R., Wilson, D., & N'jie, N. (2013). *Investing in communities achieves results: Findings from an evaluation of community responses to HIV and AIDS. Directions in development: Human development*. World Bank.
Ross, M. W., Nyoni, J., Ahaneku, H. O., Mbwambo, J., Mcclelland, R. S., & McCurdy, S. A. (2014). High HIV seroprevalence, rectal STIs and risky sexual behaviour in men who have sex with men in Dar es Salaam and Tanga, Tanzania. *BMJ Open, 4*, e006175.
Semugoma, P., Beyrer, C., & Baral, S. (2012). Assessing the effects of anti-homosexuality legislation in Uganda on HIV prevention, treatment, and care services. *SAHARA-J: Journal of Social Aspects of HIV/AIDS, 9*, 173–176.
Stahlman, S., Beyrer, C., Sullivan, P. S., Mayer, K. H., & Baral, S. D. (2016). Engagement of gay men and other men who have sex with men (MSM) in the response to HIV: A critical step in achieving an AIDS-free generation. *AIDS and Behavior, 20*(Suppl 3), 330–340.
Strand, C. (2011). Kill Bill! Ugandan human rights organizations' attempts to influence the media's coverage of the Anti-Homosexuality Bill. *Culture, Health and Sexuality, 13*, 917–931.
Tamale, S. (2009). A human rights impact assessment of the Ugandan anti-homosexuality bill 2009. *The Equal Rights Review, 4*, 49–57.
Tanzania Commission For AIDS. (2013). *Tanzania HIV/AIDS and Malaria Indicator Survey 2011-12*. Tanzania Commission for AIDS (TACAIDS), Zanzibar AIDS Commission (ZAC), National Bureau of Statistics (NBS), Office of the Chief Government Statistician (OCGS), ICF International.

The Citizen. (2019). *Tanzania: Board revokes six NGOs' license*. Retrieved July 6, 2019, from https://www.thecitizen.co.tz/News/Tanzania%2D%2DBoard-revokes-six-NGOs%2D%2Dlicense/1840340-5079110-ruc0iqz/index.html

The Prime Minister's Office. (2003). *The national multi-sectoral strategic framework on HIV/AIDS 2003–2007*. Tanzania Commission for HIV/AIDS.

UNAIDS. (2016). *Investing in community advocacy and services to end the AIDS epidemic*. Retrieved October 11, 2019, from https://www.unaids.org/en/resources/presscentre/featurestories/2016/april/20160404_community_advocacy

UNAIDS, & Stop AIDS Alliance. (2015). *Communities deliver: The critical role of communities in reaching global targets to end the AIDS epidemic*. Retrieved July 6, 2019, from https://www.unaids.org/sites/default/files/media_asset/UNAIDS_JC2725_CommunitiesDeliver_en.pdf

United Republic of Tanzania. (1998). *Sexual offences special provisions act*. The Government Printer. Retrieved October 11, 2019, from https://www.ilo.org/dyn/natlex/docs/ELECTRONIC/67094/63635/F532037758/TZA67094.pdf

Wade, A. S., Kane, C. T., Diallo, P. A., Diop, A. K., Gueye, K., Mboup, S., et al. (2005). HIV infection and sexually transmitted infections among men who have sex with men in Senegal. *AIDS, 19*, 2133–2140.

World Health Organization. (2014). *Consolidated guidelines on HIV prevention, diagnosis, treatment and care for key populations*. World Health Organization.

Chapter 6
Moral Panic and Other Unintended Consequences in Ghana's Paradigm Shift to Address HIV Among Men Who Have Sex with Men

Akua O. Gyamerah

In 2011, Ghana made a historic shift in its national HIV response by including men who have sex with men in the 2011–2015 HIV National Strategic Plan for the first time, marking a paradigm shift. This chapter examines how the criminalization and stigmatization of male same-sex sexual activities have shaped HIV prevention and care activities within this new paradigm. It explores how the legal and social context has informed and constrained HIV stakeholders' response to the epidemic among men who have sex with men and discusses the unintended consequences of prevention and care activities within the new paradigm. Through an analysis of social, political and media developments, it demonstrates how approaches and initiatives to address HIV among men who have sex with men have contributed to the politicization of homosexuality in Ghana and reshaped the context in which stakeholders develop and implement HIV policies and programs for members of this population.

6.1 "Heterosexual Africa": An HIV Policy Blind Spot in Africa

As in many parts of the global North, there exists significant HIV disparities in African countries between men who have sex with men[1] and the general population. In sub-Saharan Africa, HIV prevalence is 13.7% among men who have sex with men

[1]Throughout this chapter, I use the term "men who have sex with men" and "queer men" interchangeably to refer to gay, bisexual and other men with same-sex desires, or who engage in same-sex sex. "Men who have sex with men" is a public health term commonly used in the global HIV response to distinguish sexual identity from sexual behavior; however, I use the term critically

A. O. Gyamerah (✉)
University of California, San Francisco, San Francisco, CA, USA
e-mail: akua.gyamerah@ucsf.edu

T. Sandfort (ed.), *Male Same-sex Sexuality and HIV in Sub-Saharan Africa*, Social Aspects of HIV 7, https://doi.org/10.1007/978-3-030-73726-9_6

compared to 1.4–6.7% among all adults (UNAIDS, 2019). Although nowadays there is awareness of the elevated HIV burden among queer men in Africa, for the first 25 years of the epidemic, leading researchers, policymakers, and development agencies described Africa's epidemic as largely heterosexual in character (Epprecht, 2008; Israel et al., 1998; Quinn et al., 1986). For HIV researchers, funders and advocates, the epidemiological data that initially emerged from the HIV epidemics in Africa suggested that HIV was heterosexually transmitted and not through same-sex sexual practices.

This construction of "heterosexual Africa" (Epprecht, 2008) created a global policy blind spot that excluded HIV transmission between men as a feature of the African epidemic. Due to the downstream effects of global policy and funding, there was a related gap in global and local policies and research, and thus in prevention and care addressing HIV among queer men in Africa (Johnson, 2007; McKenna, 1996; Parker et al., 1998; Reddy et al., 2009).

6.2 A Paradigm Shift to Key Populations

Over the past decade, an increasing number of African governments have begun to acknowledge and address HIV among queer men. By 2013, more than two-thirds of African National Strategic Plans (NSPs) on HIV made mention of "men who have sex with men" (Makofane et al., 2013)—a proportion that increased by 25% five years later (World Health Organization, 2018). The change marked an HIV policy paradigm shift from *a general population* to *a key populations paradigm* (Gyamerah, 2017).[2] Key populations, according to the World Health Organization (2018), are populations who are at higher risk for HIV who face social and legal challenges that increase their vulnerability. They include sex workers, men who have sex with men, transgender people, people who inject drugs, and people in prisons and other closed settings (*ibid*, p. 4).

The key populations paradigm may be understood as a type of biopolitical paradigm—that is, an array of local and international HIV policy frameworks, priorities, and objectives, as well as programmes and initiatives, that identify criminalized and marginalized populations (i.e., key populations like men who have sex with men) as at high risk of acquiring HIV and thus, the subjects of biomedical and state interventions in the HIV response (Gyamerah, 2017). Beyond the legal contexts that criminalize them, queer men within this policy paradigm are

and share the concerns raised by scholars and activists about the limitations and reductive effect of the term's use (e.g., Kaplan et al., 2016).

[2]This chapter is based on sections of a doctoral dissertation, "Unburying the Ostrich's Head and Opening Pandora's Box: A Paradigm Shift to address HIV among Men who have Sex with Men in Ghana's National AIDS Response", (Gyamerah, 2017).

acknowledged as a legitimate group in need of HIV services—a process that medicalizes and further politicizes male same-sex sexualities.

The paradigm shift to address HIV among queer men is an important development in Africa that offers hope for the future of HIV prevention and ultimately, its elimination. By identifying this group as a population at-risk for HIV, more resources are allocated to prevention and care. However, there have also been unintended consequences of this shift in HIV policies in contexts where same-sex practices between men are criminalized and stigmatized, which must be examined to understand their impact on, and implications for, HIV prevention and care among queer men in Africa.

6.3 Ghana as a Case Study

In this chapter, I use Ghana's 2011 HIV policy paradigm shift as a case study to examine (1) how criminalization and sociocultural stigma against homosexuality have shaped key stakeholders' approaches to including men who have sex with men as a key population in the HIV response; and (2) how the new paradigm and initiatives have contributed to and been affected by unforeseen developments and moral panics related to criminalization and sociocultural stigma against homosexuality. In particular, I discuss three key approaches stakeholders have taken in Ghana's HIV policies and programmes for men who have sex with men due to the pressures exerted by the legal and sociocultural context: (1) constructing men who have sex with men as posing a risk, (2) hesitating to adopt a human rights framework, and (3) using a discreet strategy to address HIV in this group. I demonstrate the limitations of these three approaches by examining how a series of local and international developments have catalysed public moral panic around homosexuality. The impact of this panic on HIV programmes is described, as well as how stakeholders' responses have been shaped by the three approaches. I conclude by identifying lessons to addressing HIV among men who have sex with men within contexts such as Ghana where sexual activity between men remains criminalized.

The Ghana case study[3] was part of a year-long qualitative study conducted between 2013 and 2014 in Accra, Ghana on the country's HIV policies and programmes for men who have sex with men (Gyamerah, 2017). The chapter reports findings from 43 interviews with state and non-state policymakers, HIV service providers, civil society organization staff, and queer men; and group interviews with 18 queer peer educators; content analysis of HIV policy and research documents, and Ghanaian media coverage of homosexuality from 2010 to 2014; and participant

[3]The study examined why and how Ghana decided to include men who have sex with men as a key population in its national AIDS policies and programmes; what cultural, social, and political factors have affected the development, implementation, and reception of these policies and programmes; and how men who have sex with men experienced these policy and programmatic efforts as well as living in a country that criminalizes and stigmatizes same-sex sexual practices.

observation of government policy work groups and local human rights, HIV, and LGBTQ community service organizations and events.

6.4 The HIV Epidemic in Ghana

Since the first HIV cases were identified in 1986, overall HIV prevalence in Ghana has varied between 1.5 and 3.6% (Ghana AIDS Commission, 2005, 2010, 2016). The U.S. President's Emergency Plan for AIDS Relief (PEPFAR, 2017) characterizes Ghana's HIV epidemic as a low-level generalized epidemic, with a national prevalence of 1.6%, mixed with a concentrated epidemic among key populations. Ghana's most recent NSP identifies "men who have sex with men" as a key population, together with female sex workers, prisoners and people who inject drugs (Ghana AIDS Commission, 2016). A 2014 Modes of Transmission (MoT) study found that 72.0% of new adult HIV infections were among general low-risk populations, while 28.0% were among key populations and their sexual partners (Ghana AIDS Commission, 2014). Men who have sex with men had the highest HIV prevalence among all populations at 18.0% and the second highest HIV incidence among key populations (Ghana AIDS Commission, 2014, 2016). Despite the high prevalence, less than half have ever tested for HIV and only 3.5% are linked to treatment (UNAIDS, 2019; Gyamerah et al., 2020).

6.5 Ghana's Paradigm Shift and Programmes for Men Who Have Sex with Men

Prior to 2011, Ghana's national policies focused on heterosexual and parent-to-child transmission as drivers of the HIV epidemic, with an emphasis on female sex workers, pregnant women, and children/youth as vulnerable populations (Ghana AIDS Commission, 2005). In 2011, however, the Ghana AIDS Commission (GAC) established a Key Populations Technical Work Group Steering Committee (KP TWG) to develop policies and coordinate HIV prevention and care for key populations. This committee consisted of state (government agencies such as the GAC, the National AIDS/STI Control Programme, the Commission on Human Rights and Administrative Justice, and prisons and police agencies) and non-state (bilateral and multilateral funders, community-based organizations representing or servicing key populations) stakeholders.

The KP TWG developed the first set of national policy guidelines focusing specifically on key populations: the 2011–2015 National Strategic Plan for

Most-at-Risk Populations[4] (MARPs). These aimed to reach 80% of identified most-at-risk populations with a comprehensive package of evidence-based HIV prevention, treatment and support by the year 2015 (Key Populations Technical Working Group, 2011). These policies for most-at-risk populations were then integrated into the country's 2011–2015 NSP, the main body of policies that guide the country's national AIDS response. For men who have sex with men, the policy aimed to provide non-stigmatizing prevention and care along with psychosocial and clinical services.

The GAC's formation of the KP TWG and the inclusion of men who have sex with men as a key population in its 2011–2015 NSP marked a paradigmatic shift in the country's HIV response. This policy shift was a product of numerous factors. Locally, advocacy efforts by LGBTQ rights groups, such as the Center for Popular Education, Human Rights Ghana (CEPEHRG), as well as preliminary epidemiological data on HIV in men who have sex with men drew the attention of local health officials and other stakeholders. Additionally, regional groups such as Sexual Minorities Uganda and African Men for Sexual Health and Rights, as well as international organizations such as the then Global Forum on MSM & HIV and the International Gay and Lesbian Human Rights Commission, had advocated for years for the recognition of men who have sex with men in African HIV policies. In response to increasing evidence of risk among men who have sex with men, international global AIDS funders such as PEPFAR and the Global Fund to Fight AIDS, Tuberculosis and Malaria, shifted their priorities in the mid-to late 2000s to include "men who have sex with men" in the Global South, and in Africa in particular (Ayala et al., 2011; McKay, 2016). This change subsequently provided targeted funding opportunities for global South countries, like Ghana, to address HIV among men who have sex with men.

Prioritizing men who have sex with men as a key population also increased resources for research and interventions on prevention and care. These programmes include HIV testing and counselling, condom and lubricant distribution, behaviour change communication,[5] and care services provided by clinical staff trained in providing services friendly to men who have sex with men. The programmes were primarily carried out by peer educators and a small number of trained clinical staff in major cities across the country such as Accra/Tema, Kumasi, Cape Coast/Takoradi and Koforidua.

[4]Most-at-risk populations was the term used to refer to groups with the highest risk of and most vulnerable to HIV by the government of Ghana before the shift in 2012–2013 to the use of the term 'key populations', due to a change in terminology used in global HIV policies and frameworks.

[5]A public health education strategy to increase public knowledge of protective behaviours and target health behaviour change.

6.6 Criminalization and Stigmatization of Homosexuality in Ghana

This paradigm shift to include men who have sex with men in HIV policies took place in a sociocultural context that both criminalized and stigmatized homosexuality. By law, LGBTQ people in Ghana do not have any rights to protection as a population. Like many other former British colonies, the country's laws criminalize "unnatural carnal knowledge"—a legal statute with colonial roots that is treated in Ghana as a *de facto* criminalization of homosexuality. The Unnatural Carnal Knowledge code, found under Section 104 of the Criminal Code Act, 1960, criminalizes sexual intercourse with a person in an "unnatural" manner or with an animal. The Act states that unnatural carnal knowledge is to be verified through "proof of the least degree of penetration" (Government of Ghana, 2003). Thus, unnatural sexual intercourse is the term generally used to describe sex between men due to the use of the term "penetration" in the code.

This legal reality shapes and reinforces the overwhelmingly negative social perceptions of homosexuality in Ghana. In a global study, the Pew Research Center (2013) found that 96% of Ghanaian respondents believed homosexuality should not be accepted by society. A separate Pew survey (2014) reported that 98% of Ghanaian respondents believed homosexuality was immoral and only 1% found it acceptable. In community, religious and media discourses, homosexuality is commonly described as evil, ungodly, filthy, un-African, a mental illness and a disease vector. Moreover, queer men are commonly depicted as sexual predators who prey on young boys and cheat on their female partners with other men. While the term "homosexuality" is used descriptively in Western lexicon, in the Ghanaian context, the term is derogatory.

Homosexuality has been the topic of much public discussion in broadcast and print media, parliament debates, and religious sermons, due to local and international developments that have further politicized the topic (BBC News, 2011; Dankwa, 2009; Joy News, 2011). The media, in particular, have served as the most public platform for these discussions and have reported on incidents that have triggered moral outrage about homosexuality. These incidents include: the arrest of a "gay" pastor (Daily Guide, 2013), accusations that political figures are gay or support homosexuality (Joy News, 2013a, 2013b; Solomon, 2013), reports of Ghana hosting "a gay conference" (BBC News, 2006; JFM, 2006), and mob attacks against LGBTQ people (Joy News, 2012). Media coverage has been overwhelmingly negative, with headlines such as, "Same-Sex Schools: A Breeding Ground for Homosexuality" (Citi News, 2011), "Homos are Filthy" (Daily Graphic, 2011b), and "Christian Council Joins Calls to Condemn Homosexuality" (Ghana News Agency, 2011b).

International attention on African LGBT rights has also affected local discussion and debate about homosexuality. Notably, in 2013, the then President of Ghana, John Dramani Mahama, became the target of public scrutiny after the media reported on his personal relationship with Andrew Solomon, a gay US philanthropist and writer. Mahama's critics claimed he would push a "gay agenda" under his presidency due to Solomon's alleged donation to his presidential campaign (Joy News, 2013b). The backlash against Mahama forced his office to release a statement asserting that the president did not "subscribe to" and would not "promote homosexualism in Ghana" (Solomon, 2013).

Circulated in the context of international debates on sexual rights in Africa spawned by the anti-gay Bills in Uganda and Nigeria (Epprecht, 2014), these media stories contributed to a political backlash against homosexuality in Ghana (Gyamerah, 2017). Over the past decade, homosexuality has been a political talking point used by politicians and public figures for political theatrics and point-scoring. The two main political parties, the New Patriotic Party (NPP) and National Democratic Council (NDC), have accused each other of promoting homosexuality or harbouring homosexuals in office to morally discredit the other. These debates have led to calls to further criminalize homosexuality, pre-emptively ban same-sex marriage, and arrest gay men (Gadugah, 2011; Smith, 2011).

6.7 Stakeholder Approaches to HIV and to Men Who Have Sex with Men

The legal and sociocultural situation surrounding homosexuality in Ghana provides an important context for the key population paradigm. As aforementioned, key stakeholders have taken three approaches to addressing the epidemic among queer men, each shaped by criminalization of and sociocultural stigma against sex between men. I will discuss each of these approaches below.

First, to argue for the inclusion of men who have sex with men in HIV policies, stakeholders have employed a risk narrative that constructs the population as substantially driving the epidemic and posing a risk to the general population, particularly women and young men. This construction derived from data from the first few HIV studies of men who have sex with men, which showed they were at risk for HIV. Specifically, between 2004 and 2009, three key studies revealed that male to male sex did exist in Ghana, that men who have sex with men had inadequate knowledge of HIV, and that they were engaged in sexual activities that placed them at high risk of HIV (Academy for Educational Development-SHARP, 2007; Attipoe, 2004; The U.S. President's Emergency Plan for AIDS Relief, 2012). One of these studies—the first bio-behavioural survey of men who have sex with men in Accra—found an HIV prevalence of 25% (Academy for Educational Development-SHARP, 2007). Another, the 2009 Mode of Transmission (MoT) study, indicated that men who have sex with men (8%) and their female sexual partners (1%) made up 9% of new HIV infections (The U.S. President's Emergency Plan for AIDS Relief, 2012). As one of the studies concluded, there was "active bridging between bisexual men and their women partners without protection, creating more avenues for the spread of HIV" (Attipoe, 2004, p. 6).

Findings from these studies attracted the attention of stakeholders in the GAC and NACP. They confirmed to donors such as PEPFAR/USAID the need for more funding and programmes for men who have sex with men. The initial epidemiological data was used by advocates, including funders and other stakeholders, to get political buy-in for the inclusion of men who have sex with men in HIV policies. However, as part of these efforts to elicit buy-in, men who have sex with men were constructed as a "bridge" for the epidemic to unsuspecting female partners, and thus, to the general population. This narrative is common, even though according to a 2009 MoT report, heterosexual new infections (46%) were much higher than those among men who have sex with men.

Also central to this construction of risk among men who have sex with men was the notion that members of this group were driving the epidemic. One stakeholder shared that, "We [stakeholders] realized that our epidemic is driven mostly by the [key] populations. If they realize that they play a very critical role in driving the epidemic, then if you want to put in interventions, they form a critical part to the solutions." Another stakeholder, who had formerly worked at a locally-based international agency and HIV programme implementing partner, explained that describing queer men as a bridge to the general population helped gain support from key commissioners in the government, "even if there is no acceptance." The stakeholder explained,

> What helped in the dialogue that I have conducted with many policymakers and people who used to be against [including men who have sex with men] but were won over is the fact that if we don't do anything in terms of access to health, which is their fundamental right. . .[and] we also have most of them who are involved in heterosexual activity and we have many of them who are not married within their own heterosexual activity and so you realize that there is the potential of getting a bridging population that can transmit infection into the population and to those they refer to as "innocent people" as far as [male same-sex] activity is concerned.

A second possible approach within the key population paradigm was influenced by the fact that stakeholders were cautious about taking a human rights lens to address HIV among queer men. Despite Government recognition of the group in national HIV policies, and despite the fact that these same policies acknowledge the legal context and anti-gay abuse that placed queer men at high risk for HIV, stakeholders did not advocate for decriminalization of sex between men. This was primarily because stakeholders, working in a staunchly anti-gay sociocultural context, feared political backlash if they challenged the criminal code. This concern was heightened by the fact that the GAC functions under the Office of the President. Thus, any efforts by the GAC to address anti-gay human rights abuses would be publicly interpreted as an attempt by the sitting president and his political party to promote homosexuality.

In addition to these concerns, stakeholders in the KP TWG or at the GAC had not reached consensus over repealing the law and legalizing same sex sexual practices. When policy stakeholders were directly asked whether their efforts should take a human rights or public health approach, most stated that the latter was preferable due to concern that the former might draw negative social and political attention. As one policy stakeholder explained, most people in Ghana do not generally "enjoy rights"; therefore, decriminalizing homosexuality through a human rights lens would likely be interpreted as asking for "special rights" for homosexuals leading to social uproar.

Due to this, the third approach linked to the paradigm shift took the form of a discreet prevention and care strategy. In line with this strategy, policies and programmes were presented to key stakeholders, implementing partners, service providers and queer men, but not to the general public to avoid negative attention and potential backlash. Stakeholders expressed concern that HIV programmes for queer men might be perceived as "promoting homosexuality." Such concern pressured policymakers and others to be discreet: prevention materials were distributed through LGBTQ or MSM-friendly organizations and networks, no public HIV campaigns discussed or depicted same-sex transmission, and only key members and parts of the government were made aware of what was being planned. While many stakeholder members of key population preferred this approach, the operation of these programmes "in the dark" away from public visibility made it impossible to advocate effectively for their expansion and further development.

6.8 HIV Data, Homophobia and Moral Panic

The limitations of the three discussed approaches became apparent in 2011—a year that was especially difficult for the Ghanaian LGBTQ community after a series of local and international events, including media publication of HIV surveillance data on men who have sex with men, catalyzed moral panic about homosexuality that impacted HIV programmes. The moral panic began in May of that year when *The Daily Graphic*, a state-owned newspaper with the highest print circulation in Ghana, published an article entitled, "8,000 Gays in 2 Regions; Majority Infected with HIV/AIDS" (Daily Graphic, 2011a). This article included unverified population size estimates and HIV data on men who have sex with men that derived from an ongoing Integrated Bio-behavioural Surveillance Survey (IBBSS) known as "The Ghana Men's Study".

The Ghana Men's Study was the country's "first population-based survey of HIV and STIs among men who have sex with men in Ghana" (GAC et al., 2012, p. 3). PEPFAR, through the CDC Ghana Country Office, has funded the study and GAC implemented it with technical assistance from the University of California, San Francisco. The study surveyed men in Accra/Tema, Kumasi, Cape Coast/Takoradi and Koforidua and aimed to produce comprehensive data on size estimation and HIV/STI prevalence of men who have sex with men to inform evidence-based programming (GAC et al., 2012, p. x).

Although *The Daily Graphic* was not the first media source to allege the growing presence of homosexuality, it was conceivably the first time this claim had been substantiated using information from an HIV key stakeholders' event. The article reported on a 1-day USAID-sponsored workshop on HIV/STI prevention and treatment in the city of Takoradi attended by "200 health workers drawn from the

17 Metropolitan, Municipal and District Assemblies in the Western Region" (Daily Graphic, 2011a). The article stated,

> Eight thousand homosexuals have been registered by non-governmental organizations (NGOs) in the Western and some parts of the Central regions, with majority of them infected with sexually transmitted diseases (STDs), including HIV/AIDS. They include students in junior and senior high schools (JHS/SHS), the polytechnics and workers.

The article further reported that at the event, it "came out" that in 2008, 2900 gays and lesbians had been registered in the two regions, but that the number had increased to 8000 in 2010, "with most of them testing not only positive for STDs but also for HIV/AIDS after they had undergone voluntary counselling and testing" (Daily Graphic, 2011a). The implication here was that homosexuality was growing in Ghana, and that it should be a cause for concern. The article also contained general information on HIV and STI prevention and treatment and outlined suggested behaviour change activities discussed at the workshop.

While the article professed to report on information from a USAID-funded workshop, the data it cited were incorrect: it is not true that there are 8000 Ghanaian queer men in the Western region or that most of them had HIV and STIs. The newspaper also did not identify a source for its claim about 2900 gays and lesbians. Prior to the Ghana Men's Study, there had been no size estimates of LGBTQ populations in Ghana. Thus, despite *The Daily Graphic's* attempt to frame the article objectively by claiming to report on information disseminated at the workshop, the sensationalist headline that most of 8000 gays were HIV-positive, coupled with inaccuracies in the reported data, undermined any attempt at objectivity. The actual report, which stakeholders finalized in 2012, estimated that "the prevalence of [men who have sex with men] in Ghana was only 0.48% [30,579] of the adult male population" (Ghana AIDS Commission et al., 2012). It also reported that about 18.0% of men who have sex with men had HIV. In the Western region, specifically, the report found that there were about 2000 men who have sex with men, not 8000, and that 4.7%, not "most", had HIV, the lowest prevalence among the four main sites surveyed (Ghana AIDS Commission et al., 2012).

Although *The Daily Graphic* article did not openly condemn homosexuality, reporting of these distorted statistics on HIV among gay and lesbian Ghanaians had its impact. A moral panic immediately followed the publication. For the remainder of the year, the media continued to report on the growing homosexual agenda and "growing incidence of homosexuality". Article headlines included, "Homosexuality in Ghana: Senior High Schools—The Real Hotspots?", "This Homosexuality Non-sense Must Stop", and "Homosexuality in Ghana—Beware of the Down-Low Syndrome". The airwaves were packed with calls from members of the general public voicing predominantly anti-gay opinions.

Some advocates chimed in on the debate, debunking some of the common arguments used against homosexuality, and arguing that "homosexuals have rights". Among them were respected public figures such as Professor Fred Togbor Sai, an internationally renowned medical doctor with decades of experience working in the government, who advocated that "homosexuals must be free to practice"

(Citifmonline, 2011b). Human rights lawyer, Nana Oye Lithur, also publicly defended the rights of LGBTQ people, asserting that "if we have homosexuals in Ghana, once they are human beings, they have human rights" (Citifmonline, 2011a). Despite their public defence of the rights of LGBTQ people, these public figures were later forced to respond defensively against public criticism by clarifying that they did not support "the act" of homosexuality, just the rights of the people engaged in it.

The immediate panic pressured political institutions to respond as well. The Ministry of Employment and Social Welfare (MESW) publicly stated that it was investigating "the alleged case of 8,000 registered homosexuals in the Central and Western Regions" and that it "doubted the source of data" (Ghana News Agency, 2011a). The Acting Chief Director of the MESW promised to find and take "appropriate action" against the NGOs behind the alleged registration. Notably, these criticisms did not mention USAID or GAC, the two named sponsors of the event in question, who could have addressed the ministry's concerns.

The ruling political party, the National Democratic Party (NDC), also responded to the panic defensively because the controversy surrounding the article reflected badly on its moral values. The National Patriotic Party (NPP)—their main political rival—used the news to discredit the NDC morally and politically in the lead-up to an election year. The NDC's National Youth Working Committee (NYWC) prepared a press statement calling for the editor of *The Daily Graphic*, to be "sacked" for spreading propagandistic information about the then President, the late John Atta Mills, seeking to undermine the NDC by creating "the false impression that the number of Ghanaians in the gay business is rising under... [the President]". The NYWC contested the validity of the "8,000 homosexuals" claim and suggested that the editor was paid by "the international gay cartel...to attract our young boys into the act of homosexuality" by "creating the false impression that 8,000 boys...have been bold to register as homosexuals" (MyJoyOnline, 2011).

These reactions indicated how little some government officials and agencies seemed to know about the work of GAC and other stakeholders to address HIV among queer men. It is unclear whether these officials were faking their ignorance of homosexuality in Ghana and the HIV efforts in question. However, the strategy by the GAC and other stakeholders to keep the HIV prevention and care efforts for men who have sex with men visible to some and not to others may have later contributed to another unintended backlash when political agencies, groups and figures promised to find, punish, and monitor organizations and other figures that were behind the alleged registration of homosexuals. MESW's response to the controversy provides one key example of this backlash. In a public statement, the acting Chief Director of MESW insisted, "We don't register homosexuals. The publication is shocking to us. It is unfortunate the NGOs were not mentioned. The newspaper should have done the Ministry a favour by mentioning the NGOs. Without that we would embark on a wild goose chase" (Ghana News Agency, 2011a). Another article reported that the Ministry of Education was "optimistic" that homosexuality in junior and senior high schools would "soon be a thing of the past" because of new efforts to educate youth about the "menace of homosexuality" including its health risks (XFM, 2011).

The most controversial of the statements from political figures was made by the Western Region Minister of Health and NDC politician, Paul Evans Aidoo, during a *Joy News* radio interview in response to the alleged registration of 8000 homosexuals in the region he represented. He reportedly "tasked the Bureau of National Investigations and all security agencies to smoke out persons suspected to be engaging in same sex" in the Western region (Gadugah, 2011). In response to pressure from his constituents, who had mobilized against homosexuality in reaction to the news, Aidoo was reported as stating that "all efforts are being made to get rid of these people in society" and that "once they have been arrested, they will be brought before the law." He also encouraged the social surveillance of queer men and asked tenants and landlords to report information to the police that could lead to the arrests of homosexuals in the Western region. He even reportedly asked a local health NGO to hand over the names of patients who were queer men (LGBT Asylum News, 2011).

Aidoo's comments caused an international uproar, mostly in Western countries. International LGBT organizations and Western media outlets denounced Aidoo's orders and the broader anti-gay sentiments surrounding the controversy. In October 2011, David Cameron, the British Prime Minister at the time, threatened to withhold UK aid from Ghana and other Commonwealth countries if their governments did not decriminalize homosexuality (BBC News, 2011), stressing how the criminal codes in question were based on outdated British colonial law. This threat caused another moral panic in the Ghanaian media, among the general public, and in cultural, political, and religious institutions. For weeks, there was endless media coverage of Cameron's controversial comments and public pressure on President Mills to assert Ghana's rejection of homosexuality and autonomy from Britain. In response to the pressure, President Mills, asserted, "I as president of this nation will never initiate or support any attempt to legalize homosexuality in Ghana" (Joy News, 2011).

6.9 The Impact of Moral Panic on HIV-Related Activities

The spate of anti-gay media coverage, moral panic and backlash negatively impacted HIV and STI programmes for queer men, peer educators, and other front-line workers. The Maritime Life Precious Foundation in particular, the leading community service organization serving queer men and other key populations in the Western region at the time, felt the brunt of the community-led anti-gay backlash. Peer educators and staff shared how local Christian and Muslim groups protested against homosexuality after *The Daily Graphic* article appeared. The demonstrations, according to Maritime's then programme manager, were "the first ever probably organized demonstrations against MSM and homosexuality" in the country. In addition, a community member had graffitied on a major road, "Kill all these gay guys", and local youth engaged in mob violence against queer men.

Maritime's peer educators discussed how media attention and social and religious backlash had made them more publicly visible, and thus more vulnerable to abuse. One peer educator recalled how scared he was after Minister Aidoo's statements. He remembered a presentation he made on a local radio station debunking the notion that gay men were engaged in *sakawa*—a local term used to describe fraudulent online activities to illegally acquire money. Instead of local callers responding to the content of his presentation, they instead made calls for the community to "kill that boy, arrest that boy." Due to this hostility, peer educators shared how "most of our [clients] didn't want to come to us again." Some men fled to other cities, like the capital, Accra, where HIV prevalence is 30%, and some "were sacked by their landlords." Others were beaten and/or kicked out by their parents. The backlash was so impactful that queer men became fearful of accessing HIV services. For a period, front-line workers had to halt programmes and go underground.

As a researcher working with CEPEHRG in Accra in 2011, I witnessed the impact of this moral panic on the city's LGBTQ community and organizations, including key stakeholders involved in the HIV response. During this period, CEPEHRG moved from a small office in a busy and popular neighbourhood, Osu, to a more residential, less accessible neighbourhood where they felt less public scrutiny. Despite this move, 2011 was a year of many battles for the organization. Peer educators and staff suffered harassment and received threats of violence and arson. Instead of implementing prevention programmes, much of their time was consumed by responding to these hostile attacks.

In an effort to address the backlash, CEPEHRG, under the leadership of the Executive Director, MacDarling Cobinnah, the Ghana Gay and Lesbian Association, and their allies formed the Coalition Against Homophobia in Ghana (CAHG). The coalition described itself as "a group of organizations and individuals that aims to counter ongoing attacks against homosexuals in Ghana" and that "supports the human rights of all human beings including LGBT individuals in the country" (The Coalition Against Homophobia in Ghana, 2011a). CEPEHRG reached out to potential local allies and sought advice from international agencies, including the United National Development Programme and international LGBT rights and HIV organization. The organization's staff and peer educators underwent security, media and human rights training to develop their capacity to manage and weather the backlash. From June 2011 until the end of the same year, the coalition wrote three press releases: one in response to the hostile climate against LGBTQ Ghanaians; the second in response to a public statement made by the GAC after *The Daily Graphic* article backlash; and the third in response to David Cameron's aid-conditionality statement.

CAGH released its first press statement on August third, 2011. The statement challenged the media, political, religious and social backlash against the LGBT community and sought to correct some of the main homophobic narratives promoted by these actors and institutions. The statement declared:

> CAHG vehemently denounces these types of sensationalist, unfounded, and bigoted attacks against LGBT Ghanaians, who are brothers, sisters, fathers, mothers, daughters and sons of Ghanaian families just like any other Ghanaians...Contrary to unsubstantiated and

> speculative remarks that homosexuals are "evil", "filthy", and "ungodly", LGBT people are our family members, co-workers, worshippers, taxpayers, voters, media people, pastors and lovers who deserve the same rights and protection under the Ghanaian Constitution as anyone else. . .CAHG calls on the government and the good people of Ghana to condemn the ongoing attacks and to support the rights of LGBT Ghanaians before our country becomes a pariah state like Uganda and Zimbabwe. (The Coalition Against Homophobia in Ghana, 2011a)

In addition to managing these threats, there was tension between CEPEHRG and GAC about how GAC had responded to the backlash stemming from *The Daily Graphic* article. In particular, CEPEHRG was concerned about the then GAC Director General's public statements in which she assured the public that the government was conducting surveillance of HIV and STI risks of men who have sex with men due to—in the words of a *Daily Guide* article—"the increase in gay activities". She explained,

> The work of the reported NGO that registered up to 8,000 MSM, if true, may just be a microcosm of the real situation on the ground. Activities of MSM may predispose some of them and their other heterosexual partners to HIV. It is important, therefore, to have the requisite data for planning HIV prevention and treatment interventions. (Daily Guide, 2011)

Although the statement was an attempt to assure the public that the government was addressing HIV and STIs among men who have sex with men, it nevertheless repeated some of the more stigmatizing beliefs about homosexuality to justify why the government was doing so. For instance, the Director General also argued that "it is important that all hands are on deck to reduce the number of young people who are lured into MSM." She called on parents, religious and traditional leaders, educators and NGOs working with young people to educate young males on the "dangers" of men having sex with men (Daily Guide, 2011). She additionally warned that "The MSM situation in Ghana is an issue that we cannot run away from" (Daily Guide, 2011).

CEPEHRG and other CAGH members found these statements disconcerting, particularly the suggestion that gay men lure young boys—a common argument moral crusaders employ to demonize homosexuality. Worried about the damage the GAC's statement might cause, CAGH released a press statement in October 2011 highlighting their concerns and correcting some of the stereotypes the coalition felt were promoted by the GAC statement. CAGH also raised concern about a GAC member who was also a member of the Christian Council of Ghana (CCG), a group that had spoken out at a press conference about the need to "condemn homosexuals" (The Coalition Against Homophobia in Ghana, 2011b). The statement also drew attention to homophobic statements made by President Mills, Minister Aidoo, as well as the back-pedalling of the new head of the Commission on Human Rights and Administrative Justice (CHRAJ) on decriminalizing homosexuality after she experienced a backlash. The statement asserted,

> The coalition believes the statement made by the Ghana AIDS Commission set the stage for the present homophobic attacks against gay and lesbian people who are just trying to live their lives on a daily basis like anyone else. We know of no members of the LGBT community who attempt to lure young people into homosexual behavior. We believe adults

> having sex with minors is wrong, whether the perpetrator be heterosexual or homosexual...We feel the statement issued by the Ghana AIDS Commission has been inflammatory and seriously misunderstood by the general public as giving license to gay-bashing and other forms of discrimination against members of the LGBT community. We call on the GAC to clearly state how its position has evolved on homosexuality in Ghana to give the public and the LGBT community a clear idea on their position. (The Coalition Against Homophobia in Ghana, 2011b)

In response to the tensions among stakeholders and the negative impacts of the backlash, the GAC and their partners, including PEPFAR, took a few important steps to address stigma and rights abuse experienced by queer men and frontline workers. As PEPFAR stated in the aftermath of the backlash,

> Ghana has gone through a prolonged period of gay bashing that has been fueled by the media and augmented by political and cultural leaders. In response to this seemingly hostile environment for MARP activities, [U.S. government's] current interventions are focused on reducing vulnerability across MARPs through improved legal protection, which should lead to a reduction of gender-based violence and coercion. (The U.S. President's Emergency Plan for AIDS Relief, 2012)

Some of the programmes which stakeholders later developed to mitigate social stigma and anti-gay backlashes included a human rights reporting system (Williamson et al., 2014), media and police sensitivity training, and a network of allies to key populations, known as M-Friends and M-Watchers, who provide social support and resources. These efforts have been limited in their scope, however, because they operate on a small scale and depend on external funding.

6.10 Discussion

The government of Ghana and other key stakeholders in the country's national HIV response have made significant progress in addressing HIV among queer men over the past decade. There has been an increase in the resources available to queer men and the community organizations that work with them—changes that hold much promise for improving HIV outcomes for this population in the years to come. On the other hand, there have also been some unforeseen outcomes of this paradigm shift and activities.

In particular, the media's dissemination of unvetted HIV data on queer men was a major unintended consequence of stakeholders' efforts to address HIV. As an outcome, unverified biomedical data on this population reached the Ghanaian public in ways that reconstituted the sociocultural terrain, politicizing homosexuality and constructing new meanings for being homosexual. The publication of this data and the backlash it caused took place despite stakeholders' efforts to be strategically discreet in their policy and program activities to avoid anti-gay public responses.

In addition, the recognition of men who have sex with men in national HIV policies is the only form of government recognition outside of the laws that criminalize male homosexuality. As a result, queer men are recognized by HIV policies narrowly as biopolitical citizens—citizens with rights to access sexual health services without discrimination under the key population paradigm—but who remain criminalized by the law and unprotected by the constitution. This contradictory position had an unforeseen consequence, which was the increased public visibility of queer men, leading to higher vulnerability to social surveillance, stigma, and violence without any legal protection. Moreover, stakeholders' hesitance to publicly support queer men due to concerns that doing so would draw public criticism and backlash left queer men with little support to mitigate these vulnerabilities.

The events described paralleled what appears to be a broader, although uneven, pattern of backlash related to same-sex sexualities, sexual rights and HIV prevention in a growing number of African countries, including Cameroon, Senegal, Uganda, Tanzania and Nigeria (Honan, 2017; Human Rights Watch, 2016; Makofane et al., 2014; Pierce, 2016; Poteat et al., 2011; Santos et al., 2013; Semugoma et al., 2012). The passage of the Nigerian "No Same-Sex Marriage" Act in 2014 and the major crackdowns on the LGBTQ community in Tanzania between 2014 and 2017 are two examples of an apparent pattern of social surveillance and repression of homosexuality linked to HIV prevention and care for men who have sex with men (Human Rights Watch, 2016; McCormick, 2016; UHAI EASHRI, 2015; Isaack, 2017).

Such panic is not new however in the context of HIV. The USA witnessed similar social backlash against the gay community in the 1980s. Biomedical and social responses to the onset of HIV—initially termed Gay-related Immunodeficiency (GRID)—medicalized homosexuality in that country by equating male same-sex sexuality with HIV, creating a legacy that still informs social perceptions of homosexuality and HIV today. In response to the early social meanings placed on HIV, Paula Treichler (1987) astutely described HIV as "an epidemic of signification", implying HIV was "simultaneously an epidemic of a transmissible lethal disease and an epidemic of meanings or signification" (Treichler, 1987, p. 32). As an epidemic of signification, HIV not only gave rise to a health crisis, but also triggered a social crisis whereby social and cultural meanings became attached to the disease and to the social groups it disproportionately affected.

The gay community in the USA and elsewhere was very different at the start of the epidemic to the sexually and gender diverse communities in African today, where same-sex attracted people are still on the defensive and are unevenly mobilized. Many have quickly experienced the impact of governmental and global shifts in attention to their risk of HIV, sexual health, and rights on the one hand, and social polarization and further criminalization of same-sex sexuality on the other. These experiences have made individuals and organisations more publicly visible, reshaping their experiences, social realities, and social risks.

Given this context, it is important to draw out some of the lessons the Ghana case study offers to international and local HIV policymakers and other stakeholders in Africa. First, policymakers and implementers should consider evaluating HIV policies and programmes for men who have sex with men comprehensively for their impact. This means evaluating the impact of outlined policy and programme objectives, not just in terms of condom distribution and the number of men reached, but also in terms of how interventions affect the wider social context in which they are implemented, and the unintended consequences they give rise to. Key questions to be asked include (1) how are initiatives for queer men being implemented and discussed publicly, and do such actions improve or increase the anti-gay and HIV stigma faced by this population; (2) how do queer men experience new and emergent policies and programmes and how do these initiatives impact—both positively and negatively—the social environment?

Beyond this, governments and other HIV stakeholders must re-evaluate the effectiveness of the approaches discussed here. As the GAC's response to *The Daily Graphic* controversy demonstrated, recent approaches appear to compromise stakeholders' ability to openly respond to backlash related to homosexuality and defend initiatives to address male same-sex transmission of HIV. In addition, stakeholders' reliance on a risk narrative that constructs men who have sex with men as posing a risk to others further contributes to stigmatizing social notions of the men as predators and disease carriers. Stakeholders must shift from a risk discourse to a destigmatizing discourse emphasizing the legal context, sociocultural conditions, and structural factors that render members of this key population at high risk of HIV.

Despite stakeholders' attempts to prevent them, moral panic and backlash are seemingly inevitable consequences of government recognition of a stigmatized population that they simultaneously criminalize in public policies. Rather than attempting to prevent a backlash through discreet programming and de-emphasizing human rights, it might be more effective for stakeholders to strategize how to mitigate the impact of such inevitable backlash. Suggestions include strategizing with queer men and organizations that serve them over how to increase resources and support for their community, as well as how to increase political buy-in for HIV efforts in ways that do not increase stigma against them.

A third recommendation is for state and non-state stakeholders to embrace a human rights framework that takes up the decriminalization of same-sex practices. This would address both a key structural determinant of HIV risk among queer men and a legal barrier to accessing prevention and care. A moderate step that stakeholders can take, in collaboration with the LGBTQ rights activists and organizations, is to begin discussions exploring how to advocate for the removal of unnatural carnal knowledge laws. A key part of this process will be to research how other African and diasporic nations, such as South Africa, Botswana, Malawi and Trinidad & Tobago, have taken steps to decriminalize homosexuality and/or suspend legal codes criminalizing homosexual acts.

Finally, the inclusion of queer men in national AIDS responses in the context of a highly polarized international and local debate about "African homophobia" has increased their visibility and reconstituted the social and political landscape in which they live, survive and experience life on a daily basis in the region. As countries such as Tanzania conduct sweeps against gay people (Agence France-Presse, 2017) and as Nigeria and Uganda attempt to criminalize HIV prevention efforts for queer men (Schwartz et al., 2015; Semugoma et al., 2012), stakeholders and researchers must increase research on how the shift to include queer men in national HIV policies may be influencing this social backlash and how the backlash in turn affects queer men and HIV programming. By examining both the intended and unintended consequences of current strategy, state and non-state stakeholders can identify the most effective ways to address the HIV epidemic among this key population.

Acknowledgement My sincere gratitude to study participants for their time and contributions and to my dissertation committee members for their mentorship and feedback. Thanks also to Danièle Fogel for her editing support. This research was supported in part by a grant from the National Institute of Mental Health (5F31MH102156-02; PI: Akua O. Gyamerah) and a grant by The Fulbright U.S. Student Program, Ghana (2013–2014). This work was also supported by a training grant from the National Institute of Mental Health (T32 MH19105–28; Principal Investigator: Susan Kegeles, Ph.D., to support the author).

References

Academy for Educational Development-SHARP. (2007). *Behavioral and HIV biomarker survey among men who have sex with men in the greater Accra Region, Ghana*. Accra.

Agence France-Presse. (2017). Tanzania arrests 12 for homosexuality. *Daily Nation*. Retrieved from http://www.nation.co.ke/news/africa/Tanzania-arrest-homosexuality/1066-4145864-g9g72dz/index.html

Attipoe, D. (2004). *Revealing the pandora box or playing the ostrich? A situational appraisal of men having sex with men in the Accra Metropolitan Area and its environs*. Unpublished. West Africa Project to Combat HIV/AIDS and STIs.

Ayala, G., Hebert, P., Keatley, J., & Sundararaj, M. (2011). *An analysis of major HIV donor investments targeting men who have sex with men and transgender people in low- and middle-income countries*. MSM Global Forum. Retrieved from http://msmgf.org/wp-content/uploads/2015/09/GlobalFinancingAnalysis.pdf.

BBC News. (2006, September 1). Ghanaian gay conference banned. Retrieved from http://news.bbc.co.uk/2/hi/africa/5305658.stm

BBC News. (2011, October 30). Cameron threat to dock some UK aid to anti-gay nations. *BBC News*. Retrieved from http://www.bbc.com/news/uk-15511081

Citi News. (2011, July 20). Same sex schools; A breeding ground for homosexuality. Retrieved from http://www.ghanaweb.com/GhanaHomePage/NewsArchive/artikel.php?ID=215144

Citifmonline. (2011a). Nana Oye Lithur: Gays have rights & must be respected. Retrieved from https://www.myjoyonline.com/news/homos-have-rights-they-must-be-respected-oye-lithur-declares/

Citifmonline. (2011b, June 24). Homosexuals must be free to practice—Professor Sai. Retrieved from https://www.modernghana.com/news/336332/homosexuals-must-be-free-to-practice-professor.html

Daily Graphic. (2011a, May 31). 8,000 gays in 2 regions; Majority infected with HIV/AIDS. *Daily Graphic*. Retrieved from http://www.ghanaweb.com/GhanaHomePage/NewsArchive/artikel.php?ID=209214

Daily Graphic. (2011b, June 21). Homos are filthy—Presby Moderator. Retrieved July 20, 2014, from http://www.ghanaweb.com/GhanaHomePage/education/artikel.php?ID=211727

Daily Guide. (2011, June 3). AIDS Commission monitors gays. Retrieved October 25, 2016, from https://www.modernghana.com/news/332303/aids-commission-monitors-gays.html

Daily Guide. (2013). Gay pastor shocks Tema girls. Retrieved February 15, 2014, from http://www.ghanaweb.com/GhanaHomePage/NewsArchive/artikel.php?ID=282471

Dankwa, S. O. (2009). "It's a silent trade": Female same-sex intimacies in post-colonial Ghana. *NORA—Nordic Journal of Feminist and Gender Research, 17*(3), 192–205.

Epprecht, M. (2008). *Heterosexual Africa? The history of an idea from the age of exploration to the age of AIDS*. Ohio University Press.

Epprecht, M. (2014, February 28). Opinion: Is Africa the most homophobic continent? *CNN*. Retrieved from http://edition.cnn.com/2014/02/28/opinion/uganda-anti-gay-law-marc-epprecht/

Gadugah, N. (2011, July 19). Minister orders arrest of all homosexuals. *Myjoyonline.Com*. Retrieved from http://www.ghanaweb.com/GhanaHomePage/NewsArchive/artikel.php?ID=214188

Ghana AIDS Commission. (2005). *National HIV/AIDS strategic framework : 2006–2010*. Ghana AIDS Commission.

Ghana AIDS Commission. (2010). *National HIV and AIDS strategic plan: 2011–2015*. AIDS Commission.

Ghana AIDS Commission. (2014). *Ghana AIDS Commission 2014 status report*. AIDS Commission. Retrieved from http://www.ghanaids.gov.gh/gac1/pubs/2014STATUS REPORT.pdf

Ghana AIDS Commission. (2016). *National HIV and AIDS strategic plan: 2016–2020*. Ghana AIDS Commission.

Ghana AIDS Commission, RIPS, NMIMR, UCSF, & CDC. (2012). *The Ghana men's study*. Ghana AIDS Commission.

Ghana News Agency. (2011a, June 7). Ministry to investigate report on the alleged 8,000 homosexuals in the country. Retrieved from http://www.ghanaweb.com/GhanaHomePage/NewsArchive/Ministry-to-investigate-report-on-the-alleged-8-000-homosexuals-in-the-210567

Ghana News Agency. (2011b, July 19). Christian Council joins calls to condemn homosexuality in Ghana. Retrieved from http://www.ghananewsagency.org/social/christian-council-joins-calls-to-condemn-homosexuality-in-ghana-31187

Government of Ghana. (2003). *Ghana criminal code, 1960 (Act 29)*. Retrieved from http://www.wipo.int/edocs/lexdocs/laws/en/gh/gh010en.pdf

Gyamerah, A. O. (2017). *Unburying the ostrich's head and opening Pandora's box: A paradigm shift to address HIV among men who have sex with men in Ghana's national AIDS response*. Columbia University Academic Commons. Retrieved from https://academiccommons.columbia.edu/catalog/ac:nzs7h44j2x.

Gyamerah, A. O., Taylor, K. D., Atuahene, K., Anarfi, J. K., Fletcher, M., Raymond, H. F., McFarland, W., & Dodoo, F. N.-A. (2020). Stigma, discrimination, violence, and HIV testing among men who have sex with men in four major cities in Ghana. *AIDS Care, 32*(8), 1036–1044. https://doi.org/10.1080/09540121.2020.1757020.

Honan, E. (2017, April 8). *How Tanzania is cracking down on lgbt people—And getting away with it*. Buzzfeed. Retrieved from www.buzzfeed.com/edithhonan/how-tanzania-is-cracking-down-on-lgbt-people-and-getting?utm_term=.nrJZV5ljRm#.yybmwLz85M

Human Rights Watch. (2016). *"Tell me where I can be safe": The impact of Nigeria's same sex marriage (prohibition) act*. Retrieved from https://www.hrw.org/sites/default/files/report_pdf/nigeria1016_web.pdf

Isaack, W. (2017). *Facing prosecution for challenging HIV policies in Tanzania*. Retrieved October 22, 2017, from https://www.hrw.org/news/2017/10/20/facing-prosecution-challenging-hiv-policies-tanzania

Israel, B. A., Schulz, A. J., Parker, E. A., & Becker, A. B. (1998). Review of community-based research: Assessing partnership approaches to improve public health. *Annual Review of Public Health, 19*(1), 173–202.

JFM. (2006). *Proposed gay conference still sketchy*. Retrieved from http://mail.ghanaweb.com/GhanaHomePage/NewsArchive/artikel.php?ID=109876#

Johnson, C. A. (2007). *Off the map: How HIV/AIDS programming is failing same-sex practicing people in Africa*. International Gay and Lesbian Human Rights Commission.

Joy News. (2011, November 2). Mills replies David Cameron: You can't threaten us with gay aid! *Myjoyonline.Com*. Retrieved from http://www.ghanaweb.com/GhanaHomePage/NewsArchive/artikel.php?ID=222797

Joy News. (2012). Vigilante gang in James Town mass gay assault. Retrieved September 1, 2013, from http://www.ghanaweb.com/GhanaHomePage/NewsArchive/artikel.php?ID=232494

Joy News. (2013a). Oye Lithur's appointment opposed over her "support" for homosexuality. Retrieved September 2, 2014, from http://www.ghanaweb.com/GhanaHomePage/NewsArchive/artikel.php?ID=262070

Joy News. (2013b, February 10). Andrew Solomon wants Mahama to take a lead role in promoting gay rights. *Myjoyonline.Com*. Retrieved from http://www.ghanaweb.com/GhanaHomePage/NewsArchive/artikel.php?ID=264601

Kaplan, R. L., Sevelius, J., & Ribeiro, K. (2016). In the name of brevity: The problem with binary HIV risk categories. *Global Public Health, 11*(7–8), 824–834. https://doi.org/10.1080/17441692.2015.1136346.

Key Populations Technical Working Group. (2011). *National strategic plan for most at risk populations 2011–2015: Leveraging a public health approach for universal access*. Ghana AIDS Commission.

LGBT Asylum News. (2011, August 6). Gay community fights government attack. *LGBT Asylum News*. Retrieved from http://www.ghanaweb.com/GhanaHomePage/NewsArchive/Gay-Community-Fights-Government-Attack-215732

Makofane, K., Gueboguo, C., Lyons, D., & Sandfort, T. (2013). Men who have sex with men inadequately addressed in African AIDS National Strategic Plans. *Global Public Health, 8*(2), 129–143.

Makofane, K., Beck, J., Lubensky, M., & Ayala, G. (2014). Homophobic legislation and its impact on human security. *African Security Review, 23*(2), 186–195.

McCormick, J. P. (2016, September 9). Tanzania threatens to ban groups that 'promote' LGBT rights. *Pink News*. Retrieved from http://www.pinknews.co.uk/2016/09/09/tanzania-threatens-to-ban-groups-that-promote-lgbt-rights/

McKay, T. (2016). From marginal to marginalised: The inclusion of men who have sex with men in global and national AIDS programmes and policy. *Global Public Health, 11*(7–8), 902–922.

McKenna, N. (1996). *On the margins: Men who have sex with men and HIV in the developing world*. Panos Institute.

MyJoyOnline. (2011, July 13). NDC Youth group calls for the head of Daily Graphic editor. *Myjoyonline.Com*. Retrieved from https://www.modernghana.com/news/339630/ndc-youth-group-calls-for-the-head-of-daily-graphic-editor.html#

Parker, R., Khan, S., & Aggleton, P. (1998). Conspicuous by their absence? Men who have sex with men (MSM) in developing countries: Implications for HIV prevention. *Critical Public Health, 8*(4), 329–346.

Pew Research Center. (2013). *The global divide on homosexuality: Greater acceptance in more secular and affluent countries*. Pew Research Center. Retrieved from http://www.pewglobal.org/2013/06/04/the-global-divide-on-homosexuality/#religiosity-and-views-of-homosexuality.

Pew Research Center. (2014). *Global views on morality*. Pew Research Center. Retrieved from http://www.pewglobal.org/2014/04/15/global-morality/

Pierce, S. (2016). "Nigeria can do without such perverts": Sexual anxiety and political crisis in postcolonial Nigeria. *Comparitive studies of South Asia, Africa, and the Middle East, 36*(1), 3–20. https://doi.org/10.1215/1089201x-3482075.

Poteat, T., Diouf, D., Drame, F. M., Ndaw, M., Traore, C., Dhaliwal, M., et al. (2011). HIV risk among MSM in Senegal: A qualitative rapid assessment of the impact of enforcing laws that criminalize same sex practices. *PLoS One, 6*(12), e28760.

Quinn, T. C., Mann, J. M., Curran, J. W., & Piot, P. (1986). AIDS in Africa: An epidemiologic paradigm. *Science, 234*(4779), 955–963.

Reddy, V., Sandfort, T., & Rispel, L. (2009). *From social silence to social science: Same-sex sexuality, HIV & AIDS and gender in South Africa*. HSRC Press.

Santos, G.-M., Beck, J., Wilson, P. A., Hebert, P., Makofane, K., Pyun, T., et al. (2013). Homophobia as a barrier to HIV prevention service access for young men who have sex with men. *Journal of Acquired Immune Deficiency Syndromes, 63*(5), e167–e170.

Schwartz, S. R., Nowak, R. G., Orazulike, I., Keshinro, B., Ake, J., Kennedy, S., et al. (2015). The immediate effect of the Same-Sex Marriage Prohibition Act on stigma, discrimination, and engagement on HIV prevention and treatment services in men who have sex with men in Nigeria: analysis of prospective data from the TRUST cohort. *The Lancet HIV, 2*(7), e299–e306.

Semugoma, P., Beyrer, C., & Baral, S. (2012). Assessing the effects of anti-homosexuality legislation in Uganda on HIV prevention, treatment, and care services. *SAHARA-J: Journal of Social Aspects of HIV/AIDS, 9*(3), 173–176.

Smith, A. D. (2011, July 21). Ghana official calls for effort to "round up" suspected gays. *The Independent*. Retrieved from http://www.independent.co.uk/news/world/africa/ghana-official-calls-for-effort-to-round-up-suspected-gays-2318507.html

Solomon, A. (2013, February 9). In bed with the President of Ghana? *New York Times*. Retrieved September 17, 2016, from http://www.nytimes.com/2013/02/10/opinion/sunday/in-bed-with-the-president-of-ghana.html

The Coalition Against homophobia in Ghana. (2011a, August 3). *CAGH press release on homosexuality in Ghana*. OutRight International. Retrieved from https://www.outrightinternational.org/content/press-

The Coalition Against Homophobia in Ghana. (2011b, October 4). *Ghana AIDS Commission statement on homosexuality sparks hate speeches, condemnation and threats from religious, traditional and political leaders*. ILGA. Retrieved from http://ilga.org/ilga/en/article/ncsBsgR1nF

The U.S. President's Emergency Plan for AIDS Relief. (2012). *PEPFAR Ghana country operational plan 2012*. PEPFAR.

The U.S. President's Emergency Plan for AIDS Relief. (2017). *PEPFAR Ghana country operational plan 2017*. Retrieved from https://www.pepfar.gov/documents/organization/272013.pdf

Treichler, P. A. (1987). AIDS, homophobia and biomedical discourse: An epidemic of signification. *Cultural Studies, 1*(3), 263–305.

UHAI EASHRI. (2015). *The other Tanzanians: A landscape analysis of the human rights of sex workers; LGBTI communities in Tanzania, 2015–2016*. UHAI EASHRI. Retrieved from http://awdflibrary.org:8080/jspui/bitstream/123456789/298/1/tanzaniabaseline_eng_lgbti.pdf

UNAIDS. (2019). *UNAIDS data 2019*. Retrieved from https://www.unaids.org/sites/default/files/media_asset/2019-UNAIDS-data_en.pdf

Williamson, T. R., Wondergem, P., & Amenyah, R. N. (2014). Using a reporting system to protect the human rights of people living with HIV and key populations: A conceptual framework. *Health and Human Rights, 16*(1), 148–156.

World Health Organization. (2018). *Focus on key populations in national HIV strategic plans in the WHO African Region*. Retrieved from https://apps.who.int/iris/bitstream/handle/10665/275494/WHO-AF-CDS-HIV-02.2018-eng.pdf?ua=1

XFM. (2011). *Ministry to check homosexuality in schools*. Retrieved March 5, 2014, from http://www.ghanaweb.com/GhanaHomePage/NewsArchive/artikel.php?ID=224704

The manufacturer's authorised representative in the EU is Springer Nature Customer Service Centre GmbH, Europaplatz 3, 69115 Heidelberg, Germany. If you have any concerns regarding our products, please contact ProductSafety@springernature.com

Printed and bound by CPI Group (UK) Ltd, Croydon, CR0 4YY
30/09/2026
02225470-0011